The End Is Nigh

An Insider's Guide to Old Age

Connie Leas

Contents

I started writing this book at age 88.

I better get a move on!

Introduction

I'm old. I'm also lucky to be alive. Only about 40 percent of Americans born in 1936 (my birth year) are in that fortunate cohort, one that the U.S. Census Bureau categorizes as "very old age" or "frail elderly." You need only be 65 to land in their old age category. If you're 75 and older your classification is "advanced age." I prefer different categories: "old old" for my cohort, and "young old" for the others.

I was introduced to the young old versus old old classification from a book called *The Seven Ages of Death* by Dr. Richard Shepherd, Britain's' top forensic psychologist. His job is to investigate deaths that look suspicious. On one occasion, he's asked to examine the bodies of a "very elderly" couple, looking to see if their deaths could have been a murder-suicide. In contemplating this possibility, he notes that murder-suicide is for the passionate and that old people are too busy coping to experience the sort of extreme passion required for such a violent act.

With his observer's eye, Dr. Shepherd—born in 1952—describes the "tipping point" at which we slide from young old age to old old age:

> The tipping point is hard to recognize, partly because its arrival is so gradual and partly because for some people it comes late and for others surprisingly early. Perhaps it can be defined as a loss of some, although not yet all, independence. Or as the

introduction of limitation. In this cohort, many previously busy, active people find that their lives have become curtailed through physical pain, illness or a sense of fatigue that has crept up on them over the years and which makes the arm-chair increasingly attractive.... Now in old old age, our world becomes significantly smaller. We devote much of the time to managing our failing bodies. And we start to rely on others, just as when we were children.

I think Dr. Shepherd does an excellent job of describing old old age—an age that I define as 80s and beyond. I'd chosen to read his book because I'm drawn to those that are science-related. (In college I was a zoology major. My classes included anatomy, genetics, embryology, and microbiology, for example—classes related to the human body.)

Lately, for obvious reasons, I've been reading books about aging. While I've found such books to be useful and informative, it occurred to me that many of the authors are middle-aged people—or at least not the old old. In addition, they tend to focus on one or two aspects of aging, such as biology or end-of-life care. I decided that an insider's view was needed—one that included the reality of our lives as well as the measures we take to manage and perhaps improve our diminished states. In addition to writing about my own experience, I've asked friends to contribute their stories.

Becoming one of the old old is venturing into new territory—an un-known realm full of surprises. Even though, as a young or middle-aged person, you know that someday you'll be old (if you're lucky), it still comes as a shock when it happens. I never realized it would be this hard. Or maybe I wasn't paying attention. My father died suddenly of a heart attack at age 79. My mother died suddenly too—while giving a speech at age 85. She never complained and never experienced years of disability or disease, so I was unaware of any pain or hardships she may have endured. Now I know. And now I want to write about it.

This book is about the realities of aging—how it feels; what happens to our bodies and minds; the range of fitness levels among old people; why our bodies deteriorate; ways to stave off deterioration; facing the need for lifestyle changes; dealing with the medical establishment; and making end-of-life decisions.

The realities of aging are my realities. If, like me, you're an old person, I want you to know we're in this together. If you're not an old person, I want you to be aware of what's to come and how to support the old people in your life. I also want you to know that, even if the end is nigh, we can still lead active lives that are satisfying and enjoyable. That's certainly the case for me.

Part One: The New Reality

Chapter One

It ain't for sissies

When I was in my late twenties, I heard my husband's aunt announce, "Old age is the shits!" I remember being shocked by that comment, not because of the language, but because it was something I'd never thought about. Sixty years later, her description rings true, although my own characterization is closer to Bette Davis's "Getting old ain't for sissies," or maybe Phillip Roth's "Old age is not a battle. Old age is a massacre." You'll discover this if you live long enough.

Being old is hard. Don't be fooled by images of Jane Fonda cavorting around with her elderly pals at age 87. She might be doing these things, but I feel confident that it's not easy for her either. We old people often say we don't feel old. What we really mean is that we don't feel old *in our heads*—a phenomenon called "subjective age." Feeling younger in our heads can be seen as a form of optimism—that we may see many productive years ahead of us. But our bodies feel old.

For me, the "not for sissies" expression started to ring true when I and others in my cohort entered our 80s. From my own experience and my research, I've learned the grim facts about the changes our bodies undergo as we age. The list is long. We have painful joints that are stiff and arthritic. We can't hear or see well. Our hearts don't fill with blood as easily as they did when we were younger, and our blood vessels grow rigid. Our muscles and bone density diminish. Our brains shrink. The disks between our vertebrae get thinner. Our metabolism slows and our immune systems weaken. Our skin becomes thin and exhibits new eruptions. Hair grows in unwanted places. Our eyes shrink and so do our kidneys. The lenses of our eyes thicken. Activities that we used to manage without thinking now require willful attention. We choke more than young people: like everything else, the muscles in our mouths get flabby, including the flap (epiglottis) that keeps food from going down our windpipes. Not only do our mouth muscles get flabby, but we have less saliva, something I've noticed myself. I can no longer eat fried pork rinds.

My sister, who was 90 at this writing, has this to say:

> The biggest issue for me has been *change* brought on by a bad fall, but also by the many losses that old age brings—mobility, deaths of friends and family, hearing and eyesight issues, and the end of activities that I enjoyed but can't manage because of low energy and curtailed driving. I've never minded being alone, but now I have few choices. It surprises me that I was so unprepared for the changes, never imagining that they could happen to me.

Being surprised, I think, is a common characteristic of old age. Even though I heard my husband's aunt say, "old age is the shits," I somehow never thought it would happen to me. Of course, I knew I'd get old, and I'd seen old people struggle, but I never imagined myself as the struggler.

Old age is scary. Because we're aware of our tenuous hold on health and life, we're prone to magnifying every sign of a downward slide. Is that pain in my back a sign of kidney disease? Is that fluttering in my chest the beginning of heart failure? Is my inability to remember someone's name a sign of dementia? Even if we're doing well, we worry about how our continuing decline will play out and what we should do to prepare. Our good fortune could disappear in an instant. If we have a spouse or partner, it's doubly scary. We worry that he or she will fall ill, become debilitated, or die.

Perhaps the scariest aspect of old age is the specter of dementia. Almost all of us, including me, have some degree of cognitive decline. For me, it's most noticeable when I'm trying to come up with names and words. According to the National Institutes of Health, "approximately two out of three Americans experience some level of cognitive impairment at an average age of approximately 70 years."

I can live with cognitive decline, but dementia is something else. Dementia is a broad term for loss of thinking ability that's severe enough to interfere with our daily lives. Thinking abilities include memory, language skills, problem-solving, visual perception, self-management, and our ability to focus and pay attention. About 5 to 8 percent of people over age 65 have some form of dementia. This percentage doubles every five years after 65. Alzheimer's disease is the most common cause of dementia. About 70 to 80 percent of people with dementia have Alzheimer's disease. But there are as many as 50 other causes of dementia. So, yes, old age is scary.

The Massachusetts Institute of Technology has an AgeLab. To simulate aging, they created an outfit that includes yellow glasses; a neck harness; bands around the elbows, wrists, and knees; boots with foam padding; and special gloves that add resistance to finger movements. Adam Gopnik, a writer for *The New Yorker* magazine, donned the outfit and discovered that every small task became effortful. Nevertheless, he concluded that such physical difficulties are "manageable." What bothered him most was being in a state of "perpetual aggravation."

Gopnik was born in 1956. He's yet to experience the real thing. The physical difficulties of old age may be manageable as Gopnik contends, and they may also be perpetual. But the aggravation, in my experience, isn't perpetual. It comes and goes. Gopnik was temporarily burdened with accoutrements that simulated old age, an unfamiliar experience for him. If he lives long enough, he might get used to it.

The purpose of the MIT AgeLab is to incubate new technologies and products for old people. The lab quickly learned that we are a market that cannot be marketed to, the reason being that we will not buy anything that reminds us that we are old. For example, after developing the "I've fallen and I can't get up!" neck pendant, they discovered that no one wants one. The same goes for hearing aids. Only one in ten of approximately 40 million American adults who need hearing aids use them, partly because we don't want to look old. I resist hearing aids because they seem like a lot of trouble. But that's probably a foolish attitude. Several studies have shown that hearing loss is strongly linked with dementia—a result of reduced brain stimulation, social isolation, and increased cognitive load that's no longer being provided.

We old people may not be in a state of perpetual aggravation, but we can rely on electronic devices, such as cell phones and "smart" TVs to bring it on. We call these devices "modern technology." When we were growing up, we used rotary dial phones to connect with people, listened to the radio for entertainment, and visited the library to look up information. It can be overwhelming to deal with the inevitable problems associated with our electronic gadgets. Courage and determination are required. One 88-year-old who had purchased a new phone reported, "I kept waking up during the night and thinking of the arrival of the phone as a monster coming to devour me."

It might help to know that the complex challenges brought on by these often-maddening devices can be beneficial to our brains. Michael Scullin, a cognitive neuroscientist at Baylor University, tells us, "The use of everyday digital technology has been associated with reduced risk of cognitive impairment and dementia." His studies and others have shown that old people who used computers, smartphones, and the internet did better on cognitive tests than those who avoided technology or used it less often.

Because of our inexperience and naivete, many of us have fallen for scams, most prominently the "grandparent" scam, in which a caller will impersonate a grandchild who's in some sort of crisis and is asking for money. Though my husband and I have gotten several such calls, we have not been victimized by them (we hang up). But we know people who have. In fact, one out of every 50 people who are called by a "grandchild" has fallen for the scam. Here's another one aimed at old people: my husband got a call from a man who said he was from Medicare and that he was calling because Medicare was converting from paper to plastic cards. When the man said he needed information about our cards, my husband hung up. (Medicare does not call people.)

According to *Scientific American* (October 8, 2025), financial exploitation is the most frequent form of abuse we experience. Because we are the fastest growing and wealthiest segment of the population, we are increasingly likely to be targeted by scammers. We control 65 percent of the U.S.'s total wealth and $13 trillion in home equity wealth. You increase your chances of becoming a target of scams if you live in a retirement community, with its concentration of wealthy and vulnerable old people. Annual losses from scams are estimated to be as high as $28 billion in the U.S.

I've been victimized in another way. At the time of this writing, someone hacked into my Amazon account and treated himself or herself to a generous gift card. The credit card company told us to contact Amazon. Amazon told us to contact our email provider. That's because I was unable to change my Amazon password. I couldn't change my password because I wasn't getting the necessary "verification code" emails from Amazon. I wasn't getting the verification codes because the fraudster had blocked all emails coming from Amazon to me. Of course, trying to reach a human to help me only heightened my frustration. It took many hours over the course of two days to resolve this mess. Even when problems aren't of this magnitude, our daily interactions with electronic devices are a source of ongoing frustration for those of us who haven't grown up with them. At times like these we must console ourselves: dealing with the devices is good for our brains!

A few months after that incident I received notice that it was time to renew my driver's license. The last time I renewed it was in 2020. Back then, because of Covid, the DMV simply mailed me my updated license. No such luck this time. I would have to go to their office. The DMV office I normally use was closed because of renovations, so I had to go to one I'd never been to, which is more than a half hour's drive from my home.

When I arrived, the parking lot was packed. After driving up and down its lanes a few times, I finally found a spot on a side street. When I got to the office, I found it was mobbed with lines of people everywhere. After locating the proper line, I reached the intake desk where a bored lady confirmed my appointment and let me know that she sent the number for starting the renewal process to my phone. "My phone is in my car," I said. (I use it in my car to listen to audio books.) Annoyed and incredulous, she handed me a tiny slip of paper with my number on it: F254. That's the number I had to watch for on the big screen that would tell me when and which window I should approach for the next step, which I won't go into here. You get the idea.

The DMV employees made no effort to modify their conduct to accommodate an old person like me, but at least I didn't have to take a knowledge test. In California, at least, it's not required for people over 70. I'm still wondering about that message sent by the intake lady to my phone. I never saw it. Was it a text message? An email? A special app? Maybe, five years from now, I'll find out, although by then they'll probably have changed their system, just as they had in the ten years since I'd last darkened their doors.

Because I've been working with computers for a long time, I might be somewhat less fearful of them than are others in my cohort. I began working as a technical writer in the 1980s. In my first job, I wrote on a yellow legal pad, which I then turned over to a secretary who typed my handwritten words (poor her) into a word processor of sorts. In my second job, I typed my work directly into a computer (scary!) but had to enter arcane codes to specify the style features, such as fonts and margins. Then WYSIWYG (pronounced wizzywig) came on the scene. It stands for "what you see is what you get." That new software allowed me to create a document that looked the same on the screen as on the printed version, just like today. It occurs to me that young people may have never heard of WYSIWYG.

Many of us old people have lots of free time. We're challenged to be creative and resourceful in filling our days with activities that are satisfying, fulfilling, and/or enjoyable. Shortly after I retired, I took a basket weaving class and made a few baskets, which were misshapen and sloppy. I found that I enjoyed collecting the material, but I'm too impatient and careless to create anything requiring craftsmanship. I eventually concluded that the pastime I most enjoy is writing. I like researching various subjects and organizing the results of my research. So that's what I do now: a weekly medical-related blog and, from time to time, a book.

Even though I enjoy writing as a pastime, I was ready to retire from my technical writing career: I wanted more free time and less stress. But many old people prefer to continue working. One of my friends, a college classmate, says he regrets having retired in his 60s. Two other classmates—a psychiatrist and an educational therapist—are still happily at work. My hairdresser is in her 80s. From what I can gather, if you're past retirement age and enjoy your work, it's best to stick with it.

Like most people nowadays, I also enjoy activities provided by my often-annoying electronic devices. I use my iPad for reading, research, communicating with friends, and playing games, such as Wordle and Words with Friends. I also play bridge online with a computer partner. This is supposedly good for my brain, but I have trouble remembering what's been played. Is the ace still out?

Speaking of puzzles, I have taken up jigsaw puzzling—not the digital kind. Working jigsaw puzzles is a pastime I like because it uses the pattern recognition part of my brain, a nice change from the sequential and logical thinking required for writing. In the middle of writing this paragraph, I Googled "jigsaw puzzles and the brain." Here's what I got from the National Institutes of Health, based on their studies: "Jigsaw puzzling is a...protective factor for visuospatial cognitive aging," which includes perception, flexibility, working memory, reasoning, and episodic memory. The article also mentioned that working jigsaw puzzles is a stress reducer. One psychotherapist says, "Puzzling can create a kind of structured mindfulness. Puzzles offer focused attention without overwhelm [!] and a sense of progress that feels soothing and satisfying. From a nervous system perspective, that's grounding."

I don't know if my nervous system needs "grounding," but I work on a puzzle every day from 4:00 to 5:00 in the afternoon, after which I start fixing dinner. This admission is to let you know that I'm an incredibly routinized person, possibly neurotically so. I have my daily and weekly routines and am uncomfortable deviating from them. I tried being more spontaneous once by cleaning house when the spirit moved me instead of on Friday morning. I couldn't stand it.

As I mentioned in the introduction, we octogenarians (and beyond) are lucky to be alive. Most people born in my birth year have died. My best friends from high school have died. My best friend/college roommate is gone too. Those of us still living are among the fortunate ones who, like me, have so far escaped dying from cancer, cardiovascular disease, Alzheimer's, diabetes, and pulmonary disorder—the "Big Five." In fact, according to the Centers for Disease Control and Prevention, we are rare: only about 2 percent of all 85-year-olds can make this claim. The CDC also tells us that, having reached this point, our odds of staying free and clear are good. Fingers crossed.

So here I am, now age 89, lucky to be alive and well, enjoying my life, and living independently with my husband, who's also in good health. I'm grateful. And yet, that expression, "old age ain't for sissies," while sounding jocular, refers to the grim truth: old age is scary, arduous, and painful. Given that reality, we can nevertheless view our situations as an adventure and a challenge, finding ways to ameliorate further decline with efforts to keep ourselves strong, healthy, and engaged with others.

Chapter Two

On the spectrum

Dr. Louise Aronson, author of *Elderhood: Redefining Aging, Transforming Medicine, Reimagining Life,* is a geriatrician with decades of experience treating old people in hospitals, nursing facilities, and in their homes. Because of her long-time and wide-ranging experience, Aronson has been an important resource for me in writing this book.

Aronson writes, "Old age is the longest, most varied period of our lives. Some people become frail in their sixties while others remain healthy past their centenary." From "frail in their sixties" to "healthy past their centenary": that's the spectrum within which each of us old people can locate ourselves. Looking about us, it's easy to see the wide variation in the health and fitness exhibited by others in the 65- to 100-year age range.

President Lyndon Johnson, when in his early sixties, referred to himself as an old man. He died of a heart attack at age 64. Some of my children are older than that! While I certainly don't think of my kids as old, I must acknowledge that they're gray-haired senior citizens with age-related health issues of their own. We're all in this together—just in different stages of the aging process. But my kids are "young old." I am "old old." As I said in my introduction, this book is about the old old.

Some people my age are bedridden while others compete in foot races. Our place on that health-and-fitness spectrum is a matter of luck, genes, resources, preparation, and determination. You may have seen people in their 90s running marathons. Or maybe you saw the 102-year-old French woman who is still teaching yoga, or the 80-year-old woman who completed the Ironman World Championship course. Watching them, we may find ourselves comparing our meager fitness levels to their astonishing health and stamina. We might even regard our infirmities with embarrassment, not acknowledging that such cases are miracles of biological luck rather than reasonable expectations for everyone.

My place on the spectrum is closer to the foot racers than to the bedridden. I'm one of those who fight old age, who "do not go gentle into that good night." For me, *fighting it* consists of trying to carry on as I always have, playing golf, cooking, cleaning house, and gardening—activities that, I must admit, become increasingly difficult the older I get. I also fight old age by trying to keep in shape, mostly through exercises and yoga, which I'll discuss later. But fighting it does not include doing anything to make myself look younger, such as dyeing my hair. (Incidentally, as near as I can tell, when people talk about "aging gracefully," what they mean is letting their hair go gray.) I admit to fighting the relentless decline in my physical capabilities, but I'm okay with looking like an old lady. It's who I am!

I'm reminded of a joke about narcissism that Pope Francis liked to tell—one that I came across after he died at age 88 on April 21, 2025, a few months after President Trump's inauguration. In discussing jokes, Pope Francis says, "I remember the one about the rather vain Jesuit who had a heart problem and had to be treated in a hospital. Before going into the operating room, he asks God, 'Lord, has my hour come?' 'No, you will live at least another 40 years,' God says. After the operation, he decides to make the most of it and has a hair transplant, a face-lift, liposuction, eyebrows, teeth ... in short, he comes out a changed man. Right outside the hospital, he is knocked down by a car and dies. As soon as he appears in the presence of God, he protests, 'Lord, but you told me I would live for another 40 years!' 'Oops, sorry!' God replies. 'I didn't recognize you.'"

I might be in better shape than many—maybe most—of my cohort. I can get down and up from the floor without much trouble. I can see and hear OK. I can drive—day and night. I'm limber enough to cut my toenails. I don't have any chronic diseases. I'm a congenitally happy person. But who am I kidding? My joints hurt, I've had both knees replaced, I have trouble retrieving words and names, my fingernails are doing weird things, my skin is wrinkled and covered with a variety of blotches, and my neck looks like a turkey's wattle. I not only look like an old lady, I feel like one.

I think it helps my sense of well-being that I'm not much of a worrier. For example, I didn't worry about getting Covid. During the pandemic, we continued going out and about, including shopping for necessities and playing golf. I wore a mask when required, but never wiped things down, or bought sanitizer or extra toilet paper, a common practice that I never understood. I don't worry about "hydrating" (I drink when I'm thirsty), or how much sleep I get. (Experts agree that 6.5 to 7.4 hours a night is normal, as is broken sleep. Those who sleep more than eight hours have a higher mortality rate.) I don't worry about eating saturated fat and I don't pay attention to expiration or "sell by" dates. I try to avoid doctor visits. However, if something hurts, I want it fixed! I've had plenty of surgeries to prove it.

I'm grateful to get needed care. But I don't get annual physical exams (or "wellness checks" as our medical establishment euphemistically calls them). I had my last annual checkup in 2002. On that occasion my doctor informed me that my cholesterol was high. I'm not worried about my cholesterol and am not willing to take cholesterol-lowering drugs. Because

I didn't want to argue with the doctor, I simply never went back for another checkup.

You probably get annual checkups because you think they might prevent you from becoming ill. I used to think that also. But I've learned that reputable medical organizations agree with my stance. For example, one of the recommendations of the Society of General Internal Medicine's "Choosing Wisely" campaign is "Don't perform routine general health checks for asymptomatic adults"—asymptomatic meaning you feel fine. Regularly scheduled general health checks, according to this group of doctors, "have not shown to be effective in reducing morbidity, mortality or hospitalization, while creating a potential for harm from unnecessary testing." Their conclusion was the result of studies that included nine trials of 155,899 patients.

After writing the above paragraph, I discovered a contrary opinion in *The Journal of the American Geriatrics Society*: "This recommendation [skipping annual checkups] has not been shown to be appropriate for individuals aged 65 and older." I don't care. I'm still not getting annual checkups. Most people probably disagree with me about this, especially those, like my friend Susan, who believes that an annual exam saved her life: her breast cancer and congestive heart failure were discovered (and treated successfully) because they were caught in a routine exam.

Nevertheless, as cardiologist Sandeep Jauhar says, "perhaps Americans don't require the volume of care that their doctors are used to providing." Jauhar maintains that a substantial amount of health care in America is wasteful. His reasons include doctors practicing "defensive" medicine to avoid lawsuits; a reluctance to accept diagnostic uncertainty, which leads to more tests; exorbitant prices; lack of consensus about which treatments are effective; and the pervasive belief that newer, more expensive technology is always better. Doctors themselves admit that 15 to 30 percent of health care is probably unnecessary.

While I don't get annual checkups, I do run to the doctor to fix painful parts. In the last four years I had both knees replaced, as well as surgery to fix carpal tunnel syndrome in both hands, plus a laminectomy to treat sciatic pain—a procedure to remove the bit of vertebral bone that was pressing on my sciatic nerve. It worked beautifully! Even so, studies suggest that up to 20 percent of surgeries in some specialties are unnecessary. The list includes repairing meniscus tears, spinal fusion, shoulder surgery for impingement (removing a bit of bone from the outer end of the shoulder blade where the arm bone "impinges"); coronary stenting (placing a tube inside an artery to open it up); ruptured Achilles' tendon surgery (wearing a boot works just as well); many fracture surgeries (if the bones are roughly aligned, they will heal themselves). There are many more.

My principal source for the above information is Ian Harris, MD, PhD—an Australian orthopedic surgeon and professor of orthopedic surgery who directs a research unit that focuses on surgical outcomes. He admits to performing surgery that doesn't work. "Sometimes," he says, "if a patient complains enough, one of the easiest ways of satisfying them is to operate." The title of his book is *Surgery, the Ultimate Placebo.* If we expect a treatment to work, it is more likely to be perceived as working. As the book blurb says, "For many complaints and conditions, the benefits from surgery are lower, and the risks higher, than you or your surgeon think." Dr. David Kallmes of the Mayo Clinic believes that doctors continue to do some of these operations because insurers pay and because doctors remember patients who seemed better afterward. As Kallmes notes, "I think there is a placebo effect not only on patients but on doctors."

In addition to maintaining or improving our physical health, it's important to pay attention to our mental health, of which connecting with others plays a significant part. These days, we're hearing more on the topic of loneliness, especially among the elderly. Typically, the media pronouncements are similar to those that I garnered from an AI query: "Loneliness in the elderly is a widespread problem with serious health consequences, linked to factors like living alone, the loss of loved ones, chronic illness, and sensory impairments." A third of all Americans over 65 live alone. A four-year study pf 41,000 people conducted by the University of British Columbia found that participants, when presented with a list of more than 80 activities, consistently rated the activities as more enjoyable when done with at least one other person—even reading quietly with strangers. "Group meals provided the biggest happiness boost."

Recently, a friend told me about Death Café. It's a worldwide organization of over 20,000 discussion groups across 93 countries. Their objective is "to increase awareness of death with a view to helping people make the most of their (finite) lives." My friend, who has since died, was quite enthusiastic about his discussion group and stressed that the gatherings are not grim and are attended by people of all ages. The organization stresses that it is not a grief support or counselling session.

I mention it here partly because I thought you might be interested and partly because it offers an opportunity to meet with others. As one woman commented about a meeting she attended, "We had 14 people at this Death Cafe.... Linda facilitated one group and David facilitated another. One table discussed the role of a death doula, the uncertainty of life, the challenges of deciding how much to involve children when a grandparent or parent is dying, how a child's experience with death at a young age can affect them decades later—among other topics." You can search for Death Café on the internet to find one near you.

I'm fortunate to be a member of a Zoom group whose members are from the Pomona College class of 1958—115 of us in that year (including

Kris Kristofferson). At the beginning of the pandemic, in early 2020, one of our enterprising and thoughtful classmates came up with the idea of gathering us together in Zoom meetings. He, along with some others, planned the first meeting and used our class listserv to invite us—about 60 people that year. (A listserv is an email address that allows cross-communication between a group of people.) We have been meeting monthly ever since—five years at this writing. Monthly attendees include classmates living in Australia and Panama.

Each Zoom meeting consists of a presentation, followed by a group discussion. Sometimes the presenters are classmates who prepare talks on their own experiences, such as running a coffee plantation in Panama, or pleading cases at the Supreme Court. Other presenters are "outsiders," giving informative talks such as "artificial intelligence in today's classrooms," or "Frances Perkins, the mother of Social Security."

I'm on the committee to plan the meetings. There are nine of us. Committee members live in California, Florida, Maryland, and North Carolina. The committee meets on Zoom once a week for an hour. It's always a pleasure to be together, even when we don't accomplish much. Our monthly Zoom meetings of about 30 attendees help to combat that loneliness and keep us connected to one another. Because our graduating class was small, we remember our fellow classmates and even recognize one another after more than 65 years. Here we are, together again!

At the same time, though, our gatherings make us aware of the precariousness of this stage in our lives as well as the variations in fitness and health among our classmates. In our five years of meeting, some attendees have died, and some spouses have died. Some have moved from independent living to retirement or care facilities. Many, including committee members, have been in and out of the hospital. Some have significant loss of sight and hearing. Some have joined us from their beds. But as we get together once a month, we smile and laugh, have lively discussions, and share news of our lives. In other words, our Zoom attendees, now all age 89, are a microcosm of our cohort—people all over the spectrum.

If you're an old person and feel more akin to the bedridden than the marathoner, it's not too late to improve your place on the fitness spectrum. While I generally don't believe in giving advice, I do feel strongly that the most important thing you can do is **exercise**. It will improve your overall health and lessen your chances of falling. This book's chapter on exercise includes examples of people in their 90s whose exercise routines are doing just that.

Chapter Three

Falling

Old people fall a lot. In the U.S., falls are reported every year by more than 14 million people over the age of 65. We get lots of advice about preventing falls, and for good reason: falls are the most common cause of traumatic brain injuries, and they're the leading cause of injury for older adults. Because of a fall, about three million old people visit the emergency room every year and about one million are hospitalized. Not only are old people injured from falls, but we die from them, and the number of deaths is increasing. Nine people I know have fallen in the past year—some multiple times. Nearly all required medical attention (none died).

For these reasons, and maybe more, when you visit the doctor's office, the medical personnel are required by the Centers for Medicare and Medicaid Services to ask if you've fallen in the last six months. The Center gathers this data to track the proportion of its enrollees who have been assessed by the doctor's office for their risk of falling. This information is tied to reimbursement. The greater the proportion of patients queried, the better the reimbursement.

Even though I don't get annual checkups, I was asked about falls by my healthcare conglomerate when making an appointment to get an EKG prior to one of my surgeries. Included in their confirmation email was a question asking whether I'd fallen in the last six months. I clicked the "No" option, which was a lie. In fact, I'd had a spectacular fall.

Here's how it happened: at about three in the morning, I remembered that we'd left a pot of chili on the stove, letting it cool before putting it in the refrigerator. I got up and went into the kitchen without turning on the light. As I proceeded toward the stove, I smashed into the corner of the dishwasher door, which had been left open. It punctured a hole in my right lower leg and sent me flying onto the hard tile floor. I landed on my right hip and twisted my left knee. My first thoughts were of houseguests who were arriving that day, and of the golf game planned for the day after that. My next thought was "this is the beginning of the end."

Then, as I lay there, it seemed that maybe I was OK. I got up off the floor, put the chili in the refrigerator, limped to the bathroom, and bandaged the puncture, which had bled quite a bit. I attribute the fact that I hadn't broken any bones to luck. That is, I probably have genes that confer dense bones. I attribute the fact that I could get up off the floor to my exercise regimen, which includes a focus on strengthening my butt and thigh muscles. I lied on the medical form because I figured that fall didn't count. I've never fallen because of losing my balance and I didn't this time. I concluded that smashing into the dishwasher door doesn't count as a real fall—I tripped! Besides, admitting to a fall might trigger a cascade of medical tests. Just leave me out of it!

Aside from tripping over impediments, old people mostly fall because we lose our balance and are unable to right ourselves. The reasons for this are various. A big one is sarcopenia, which is a decline in muscle mass, strength, and function. In addition, as we age, our peripheral nerves become less effective, which reduces our body awareness, thus making it harder to recover if we start to wobble. Other reasons include problems with balance and gait; blood pressure that drops too much when getting up (postural hypotension); failing eyesight, hearing, and reflexes; conditions such as diabetes, heart disease, or problems with our thyroid, nerves, feet, or blood vessels; cognitive impairment or certain types of dementia; foot problems; and side effects of medications (the more medications you take, the more likely you are to fall, as discussed in the next chapter).

Falling is especially dangerous for people (mostly women) who have osteoporosis, a disease that causes bones to become weak and brittle, making them break easily in a fall. (Osteoporosis means "porous bone.") According to the National Osteoporosis Foundation, about 20 percent of women aged 50 and older in the U.S. have osteoporosis. At age 80 that number increases to about 40 percent. Over 300,000 people are hospitalized every year because of hip fractures. Of those, 20 percent will die within one year. If I had osteoporosis, my nighttime fall on the kitchen floor would most likely have resulted in at least one broken bone.

Interestingly, studies have shown that fear of falling can be a risk factor itself. People who are afraid of falling often walk slowly and stiffly, thus increasing their chances of taking a fall. Their rigidity makes it harder to make a quick recovery step. Those with osteoporosis are especially—and understandably—afraid of falling. Their fear often leads them to restrict their activities and become less mobile, thus making matters worse: they create a self-perpetuating cycle of inactivity and increased fall risk.

To prevent falling, we old people need to build strength and balance by doing exercises that build up our butt and thigh muscles, such as sit-to-stand exercises—basically standing up from a sitting position. A good way to do this is to stand in front of a chair, then, keeping your heels glued to the ground, bend your knees and slowly, through a count of five, lower yourself until your buttocks gently touch the chair seat. Try not to actually sit. Rise from the chair and straighten your legs through another count of five.

Here's what else you can do: rather than buy a raised toilet seat or install grab bars next to your toilet, train yourself to get up off the toilet without using your hands. It's what I do. The muscles you use to do this are those that keep you from falling.

A variety of fall prevention programs are available online, such as those offered by AARP or The National Institute of Aging. Because falls often happen when you stand up and turn, performing tai chi is a good way to practice turning safely. One researcher, a physical therapist, observes that many old people walk pitched forward with shuffling feet. She recommends walking with Nordic walking poles which encourage a slight rotation of the arms each time a pole is planted, a move that improves stability.

Friends who live in a retirement community tell me that, when residents fall, they are asked if they've hit their heads. If the answer is yes, they are taken to the hospital to be checked for possible brain injury. If the injury is severe, the person may have a life-threatening brain hemorrhage. But this is unlikely. If anything, he or she might have a concussion. *Concussion* is another word for mild traumatic blunt injury. Hitting your head can transmit a wave of pressure through the brain that can temporarily stun the neurons. Any damage to the brain caused by a concussion cannot be detected by a CAT scan or MRI. That's because the damage occurs on a microscopic level. For this reason, a diagnosis is based on symptoms: headache, sensitivity to light, dizziness, nausea, vomiting, and amnesia. (With most concussions, there's no loss of consciousness.) Such symptoms can last anywhere from seconds to weeks or even months.

Some assisted living facilities have installed fall-detection systems—sensors mounted high on the wall or on the ceiling that capture the movements of people in the room. If a resident falls, the sensor alerts the building staff to come immediately. Some sophisticated sensors monitor gait, posture and patterns of movement. Using predictive analytics, sensors learn the trends that can portend a fall—information that can be used to help prevent future falls and that has, in fact, reduced falls in the facilities that use them.

Reviews of monitoring systems have been mixed. For example, in response to the sophisticated system in one facility, the sister of a resident writes: "The system has been a godsend...she had one fall in the past year. Before that, it was every four to six weeks." In response to the less sophisticated system, one reviewer writes, "My wife is in a facility with such a system. It does not prevent falls. At best, it provides faster response to falls that occur. Staffing levels limit the ability of facilities to respond to the alerts."

From what I can gather, firefighters are the go-to group for dealing with falls. I asked my neighbor, Will, who is a firefighter, about his experience in dealing with old people who have fallen. He tells me that sometimes all that's needed is a "lift assist," but that other times the fallen person also needs medical attention. In Will's experience, the firehouse gets called to a lift assist about two times during every shift, although he's been known to respond to as many as five times in a single shift. Of these calls, depending on the fire district's location, about 50 to 75 percent come from assisted living or nursing homes. Typically, he tells me, the falls are precipitated by "medical conditions leading to generalized weakness, lack of coordination, instability, and dizziness related to the use of anti-hypertensives or narcotics." If the person was alone and incoherent when found, the cause of the fall may remain unknown.

Firefighters take a fire engine to the scene along with an ambulance if required. Once there, they help the fallen person into a chair or bed or to the restroom, if needed. Before leaving, they check the surroundings for impediments that might precipitate another fall. They also ask questions to ensure that nothing more is needed from them and to determine frequency of falls. (Some calls for help come from "frequent flyers," people who fall on a regular basis and who are familiar to the firefighters. Statistics have proven that a single fall increases the probability of more falls.)

In a home situation, firefighters are called because family members are unable to lift the fallen one. A person living alone can be on the floor for hours or days before he or she is discovered. In a nursing home or assisted living facility, Will says, "the aides typically do have the capacity to lift the patient but seek the muscular aspect of the fire department. It's easier to call us and have two of us lift the patient than three of the staff lifting the patient."

A person is transported to the hospital if it's obvious that a higher level of care is required, as indicated by signs of trauma such as loss of consciousness and abnormal bleeding. Hospitalization may also be required if the responders find signs of stroke or disorientation or deviations from the fallen person's "baseline status" as determined by information in past medical history, such as high or low blood pressures, or EKG anomalies. Sometimes, the patient requests to be transported to a hospital, and sometimes one of the firefighters will ride in the ambulance to assist the paramedics.

In Omaha, Nebraska, the fire department noted that they were called for a lift assist nearly every day by an assisted living or nursing facility. On arrival, they'd find no medical emergency or injury. They also noted that the calls increased as the facilities reduced staffing, especially in the evenings and weekends. After introducing a $400 fee for these calls, their numbers fell significantly.

I learned that you can buy inflatable lifting cushions to help get a fallen person off the floor. The devices come in various styles and prices. To use the devices, you must somehow get the person onto a deflated cushion—perhaps by rolling them—then inflate it. After searching for lifting cushions on my computer, I found the "Joerns Mangar Supine Transfer System with Airflo Duo and Bag" for $8,000. More typical is the "HelpUp Patient Lift" for $400.00. I watched a video of one of these gadgets. The video didn't include the part about getting the person from the floor onto the deflated cushion. That's the part I wanted to see. In imagining this effort, it strikes me that calling the fire department would be the easier and cheaper solution.

By starting a regimen of exercises, you can prevent falls, or, if you do fall, you'll be able to get yourself up off the floor. I do this. There's nothing special about me. I'm an old lady. If I can keep myself from falling and can get up off the floor, so can you.

Chapter Four

Polypharmacy

Drugs can increase the risk of falls. Old people who take four or more prescriptions a day are 1.5–2 times more likely to experience recurrent falls than those who do not. Taking that many pills in a day is called *polypharmacy*, a regimen practiced by one in five U.S. adults.

According to Dr. Thomas Farley, an epidemiologist, the biggest culprits in causing falls are those drugs that make you drowsy and/or that act on the central nervous system, such as benzodiazepines (e.g., Xanax and Ativan), opioids, antidepressants, and gabapentin. But other drugs, such as anti-hypertensive drugs for high blood pressure are also responsible for falls. As reported in *The New York Times*, one man had been taking a drug (Xtandi) for his prostate cancer off and on for four years. "It seemed like I was falling every other month. It was kind of crazy." After he stopped taking the drug, he reported, "I haven't had a single fall since."

I occasionally take over-the-counter pain medications for my arthritis, but no prescription medications, so polypharmacy is not an issue for me. But it is a problem for many old people. In fact, a recent article in *JAMA Open Network* states that 45 percent of adults over 65 are "exposed to polypharmacy." The older the patients, the more likely they're taking even more than five medications.

The problem with taking so many drugs is that they can have adverse effects, which increase exponentially if you're on four or more medications. In addition to a greater risk of falls, studies have shown that polypharmacy is also associated with a faster decline in memory, excessive bleeding, dangerously low blood sugar, and other complications. Drugs are the most common cause of delirium.

More than 6 percent of all hospital admissions are because of adverse reactions to medications. For people over 65, it's more like 12 percent. Even more alarming is the FDA statement, "adverse drug reactions are one of the leading causes of morbidity and mortality in health care." Prescription drugs, even when properly prescribed, rank fourth, along with stroke, as a leading cause of death. About 128,000 people die every year from drugs prescribed for them, and that number is rising sharply.

The reasons for the high mortality rate are the high prescription rates. In 2016, over four billion prescriptions were filled in the U.S. That's about 12 prescriptions for every person in the country. Sixty-four percent of all visits to physicians result in prescriptions (this was in 2000; it's probably much more now).

Being an old person makes you a target for the pharmaceutical industry. When Medicare added drug coverage, in 2006, pharmaceutical companies increased their advertising, especially in areas with a high proportion of residents over 65.

Geriatrician Dr. Louise Aronson, says, "it's likely that [symptoms of illness] caused by drugs are never diagnosed. In a healthcare system where time is the scarcest resource and care is fragmented among doctors...new symptoms are too often attributed to age and disease rather than to the drugs that actually caused them."

Just because a drug has been approved by the FDA doesn't mean it's safe. Even after a drug has been approved, the risk of serious adverse reactions is one in three. The most infamous example was Vioxx, an FDA-approved drug which experts say caused about 120,000 traumatic cardiovascular events and 40,000 deaths. The drug is no longer on the market.

Even aspirin has risks, and those risks, which include internal bleeding, hospitalization, and death, increase considerably with age. A 2011 study found that aspirin was one of the top four drugs associated with emergency hospital visits in people over 65. A dear friend of mine, who has died, went to the doctor complaining that she was gasping for breath at the slightest exertion, such as walking upstairs. She also had blood in her stool. Her doctor discovered she was severely anemic and sent her to the hospital for a transfusion. Because of having had a heart attack, she had been on Plavix, a blood thinner that is used to prevent clotting. She'd also been taking aspirin.

After she got to the hospital, the nurses quickly named Plavix as the culprit, and she was immediately taken off it. (This diagnosis of drug-induced bleeding was never formally acknowledged in written form.) My friend had the transfusion on a Friday, then languished in the hospital over the weekend waiting to be seen by a gastroenterologist. The idea was to look for ulcers, supposedly the cause of the bleeding. An endoscopy showed no ulcers. "They must have healed," the doc concluded. She saw her cardiologist a few days later. He took her off the aspirin but put her back on Plavix as a stroke-prevention measure.

On learning of her experience, I felt compelled to start researching this. Among other things, I learned that Plavix users are twelve times more likely to develop ulcers, gastrointestinal bleeding, and cerebral bleeding. For people who have had bare metal stents inserted following a heart attack, a drug regimen of Plavix plus aspirin is advised for only *one month*. Those with medicine-coated stents can be on the regimen for *six to 12 months*.

My friend, who'd had a stent inserted following her heart attack, was on this regimen *for 15 years*!

Dr. Aronson complains that medication dosages and risks don't take into consideration the aging body. "The body's response to drugs changes and the risk of drug side effects increases in old age. While precautions specify risks to children, pregnant women, and people with certain diagnoses, they do not mention possible harms to older people." Because age changes the kidney and liver, which are responsible for clearing medications from our bodies, we old people are particularly susceptible to adverse reactions.

One of the reasons prescriptions and dosages could be inappropriate for old people is that our age cohort is not included in drug trials. For example, while it's mostly older people who have atrial fibrillation, there have been no requirements to include them in trials of the drugs designed to treat that condition.

Similarly, the mean age of participants in a randomized control trial for treating osteoporosis was 64. But the mean age of people with this condition is nearly 85. As Dr. Aronson notes, "This is like studying menopause in thirty-year-old women." She tells the story of an old woman who'd developed a relatively minor and treatable problem and who'd been given a dose of a drug suitable for a middle-aged woman. The side effects of the drug landed her in the hospital, where she not only got an infection from an IV site, but also fell and broke her arm.

In her practice, Dr. Aronson often sees old people suffering from a "prescribing cascade." For example, she tells of a man who was prescribed a new blood pressure pill which caused him to have gout. Rather than changing medications, his doctor treated the gout with a strong anti-inflammatory drug that caused heartburn. "And so it went, each side effect treated with another medication that caused another side effect that was treated with yet another medication, and so on. Just as bad, even when his problems got better, as his gout had, the medications were continued. In just a few months, he'd gone from healthy to bedbound."

Dr. Aronson's book also includes an account of an elderly man who was near death and was clearly not going to improve. "That day," she writes, "we stopped his heart medications....And still he didn't die. For weeks, then months, nothing changed. It seemed he hadn't needed all those medications, something I often see."

I tend to go overboard in cautioning about drug use. I know that medicines can and do improve the quality of people's lives, not to mention conquer diseases and save lives. I'm certainly in favor of taking them when needed. As with me and my surgeries, we want our problems fixed! I have friends who would not be alive were it not for the medicines they take. I take them myself sometimes, such as antibiotics for a urinary tract infection. Recently, my husband was helped enormously by a drug prescribed for him. He had developed an auto-immune-type of disorder that left him fatigued, in pain, and curtailing his activities. The drug he took worked wonders. Almost immediately, his symptoms abated. He got his life back.

That said, I'd still recommend that, if you take multiple medications, it might be time to review them with your healthcare provider. Their side effects could be problematic.

Part Two: What the Scientists Say

Chapter Five

Aging research

Research on aging used to be a scientific backwater. That's no longer the case. Aging research has taken off, most probably because of a growing elderly population. We're beginning to experience an "age wave"—a swift and substantial increase in the numbers of us who are age 80 and above. According to the U.S. census, in 2025 alone, our numbers increased by 3.4 percent. By 2035, our numbers are expected to increase from 14.7 million to nearly 23 million, a growth rate of over 55 percent—a rate that outpaces every other age group. Of course, such demographics foretell problems, primarily because of the burdens placed on health care and Social Security—changes that contribute to financial strains on these institutions. To compound the problems, labor force shortages are also predicted. Attention must be paid.

Attention is being paid. Dozens of institutes around the world are devoted to the study of aging. Examples include the National Institute on Aging (part of the National Institute of Health), the Center for Aging and Health (Johns Hopkins), the USC Leonard Davis School of Gerontology, and the Center for Aging Studies (Delhi, India). In the last ten years alone, more than 300,000 scientific articles on aging have been published. More than 700 start-up companies have invested heavily in research to tackle issues related to our aging population. Unsurprisingly, pharmaceutical companies have also started aging programs.

Because of these studies, we know a lot about what happens to us in old age. What the studies tells us is that longevity is mostly a matter of luck. We're all aware of people who live to 100 and beyond, but such people are extreme outliers. Scientists don't know what contributed to their longevity, although it appears that they're protected by the "right" genes. Because centenarians have very little in common genetically, nobody knows what those longevity genes are. Not only are centenarians extreme outliers, their life histories and habits tend to be idiosyncratic. They're no more health conscious than the rest of us. In a study of centenarians at the Institute for Aging Research, researchers found that many of those who had reached 100 had "dubious" lifestyle habits: some were big smokers or drinkers or were unhealthily overweight. Some exercised; some didn't.

Jean Calment, thought to be the oldest person on record, died at the age of 122 (there's some debate about this, as explained in Chapter 8). She smoked for all but the last five years of her life. She ate more than two pounds of chocolate every week and rode a bike, we're told, up until the age of 100. More recently, in 2025, Maria Branyas Morera, a Spaniard, was deemed the "world's oldest person." She died at the age of 117. (I saw a picture of Maria in *The New York Times*. She looked every bit her age.) Of course, people posit all kinds of theories about why Maria lived so long: diet, exercise, healthy microbiome, close family and friends, and so forth. Scientists at the University of Barcelona's School of Medicine studied her genes and concluded that she had genetic variants that have been reported to protect against risk factors such as heart disease and cancer. Other scientists are less convinced. For example, geneticist Dr. Mary Armanios, at Johns Hopkins School of Medicine, says that "The genetics of longevity are notoriously confusing." Some geneticists believe a large, well-controlled population study is what's required.

In 2003, researchers at the University of California, Irvine, discovered a survey that had been completed in 1981 by 14,000 residents of Leisure World, a retirement community in California. In that survey, residents had provided data about their diets, exercise, vitamins, activities, and other health-related matters. The researchers discovered that 1,900 of those who'd completed the 1981 survey were still alive, so they enrolled 1,600 of them in a follow-up study. Some results were unsurprising: people who exercised and had a satisfactory social life lived longer than those who didn't. Taking vitamins had no benefit, but consuming caffeine and moderate alcohol was associated with living longer, as was having average or above average weight. Most interesting to me was the fact that those with high blood pressure had less dementia. (I have high blood pressure.)

Another area of research is body mass index (BMI), a measure of health used by healthcare professionals. (To calculate your BMI, divide your weight by your height.) According to this screening tool, a BMI between 18.5 and 25 is a "healthy" or "normal" weight. Above 25 is thus "overweight." But overweight people like me live longer than healthy-weight people! This has been well documented and is irrefutable. For example, a study that followed 1.8 million people for ten years found that people with a BMI between 26 and 28 had the highest life expectancy. The researchers also found that people with a BMI between 18 and 20 had a lower life expectancy than those with a BMI *between 34 and 36* (obese*)*. The most recent study, published in the May 2016 *Journal of the American Medical Association*, showed that people with a body mass index of 27 have the lowest risk of dying early from any cause. My BMI is 26.3 (overweight). I don't understand why we're called overweight if we live longer than "normal" people.

For 25 years, scientists have been studying super-agers, a term coined by Dr. M. Marsel Mesulam, founder of the Mesulam Center for Cognitive Neurology and Alzheimer's Disease at Northwestern University. Super-agers are people aged 80 and up who have the memory ability of a person 20 or 30 years younger. Since 2000, 290 people who met this criterion have been studied at the Center, and the scientists have autopsied 77 of their brains. Some of the brains contained amyloid and tau proteins (also known as plaques and tangles), which are known to play key roles in the progression of Alzheimer's disease, but others didn't develop any. The researchers found that super-agers' brains were either resistant to making plaques and tangles, or, if they made them, the plaques and tangles didn't affect their brains. They had resilience.

The brains of super-agers are also less atrophied than the brains of their peers: more on par with 50- and 60-year-olds. These folks are relatively rare—probably less than 10 percent of old people. Interestingly, studies have shown that super-agers don't necessarily have better health habits than others: their diets, amount of sleep, professional backgrounds, and alcohol and tobacco use weren't better than non-super agers. Some exercised regularly; some never had. As one researcher commented, they probably have "some sort of lucky predisposition or some resistance mechanism in the brain that's on the molecular level that we don't understand yet."

New research has shown that super-agers tend to be extroverted. According to neuroscientist Ben Rein, "People who socialize more are more resistant to cognitive decline as they get older. They have generally larger brains." Scientists surmise that socializing may protect our brains from atrophy, perhaps because loneliness can increase levels of the stress hormone cortisol. Increases in cortisol can lead to chronic inflammation, which can damage brain cells and increase the risk for dementia.

Then there's this: new research has also found that super-ager brains tend to have more of a special cell, called *von Economo neurons*, that are found only in highly social mammals, such as apes, elephants, whales, and humans. Such neurons help build and maintain powerful, strong social connections. The discovery of these special neurons leads to a "chicken and egg" conundrum. As one researcher noted, "Whether it's the socialization that leads to maintenance of better cognition, or whether it's the better cognition that leads to more socialization, I think is still open to debate."

For me, this degree of mental sharpness brings to mind Eric Kandel (born 1929) as well as Warren Buffet (born 1930), super-agers I have seen interviewed on television. They're never grasping for words! Kandel is a Nobel prize-winning neuropsychiatrist who did not retire from his position at Columbia University until 2022. Buffet, the well-known investor, didn't retire as chairman of Berkshire Hathaway—an international investment conglomerate—until age 95. Both Buffet and Kandel strike me as cheerful sorts.

It's likely you're not a super-ager. Neither am I. I am, however, a woman, which is in my favor in terms of longevity. Women outlive men. In the United States, we women have a life expectancy of about 80, compared to 75 for men. We don't, however, live *better* than men. We're more physically frail than men in old age and we're also more vulnerable to developing cardiovascular problems and Alzheimer's disease, but that might be because we live longer and have more opportunity to develop those diseases.

While nearly twice as many women are diagnosed with Alzheimer's disease as men, recent research has found that women's brains age more slowly than men's. We have better memories and cognitive function than men of the same age. In men, there's a greater reduction in volume across more regions of the brain than in women. For example, a large study found that the postcentral cortex, which is responsible for processing sensations of touch, pain and temperature, as well as sensing the body's position and movement, declined by 2.0 percent a year in men and by 1.2 percent a year in women. Women also have better immune systems, at least until menopause, and we practice more "health-promoting behavior," such as adhering to public health measures and avoiding risky driving.

Because we old people are increasingly becoming the objects of study, researchers are currently amassing lots of data about us—who we are, what we eat, how we live, and the states of our bodies and minds. They're also studying the causes of aging and ways to extend our "health span"—the now-popular term for the number of years we live in good health, free from major chronic diseases and disabilities. I'll deal with that in chapters that follow.

The causes of aging

As you slide from being a member of the young-old group into that of the old-old, you might become baffled by your decline. Why is this happening? Can you stop this? Can you fix it? Like life itself, the aging process is complicated. You can't stop it, but maybe you can make it less debilitating.

Most of the information in this section comes from a book titled *Why We Die*, by Venki Ramakrishnan, winner of the Nobel Prize in Chemistry. Ramakrishnan tells us that aging doesn't have one or a few independent causes. It's a highly intricate and interconnected process, one that includes the accumulation of chemical damage to our cells over time. The process starts with small defects in our complex systems. These lead to medium-sized defects, and so on. As we age, the quality control and recycling machinery of our cells deteriorates, and can lead to inflammation, neurodegenerative diseases, osteoarthritis, cancer and other pathologies.

Hundreds of scientists throughout the world are studying the processes that give rise to both aging and cancer. One structure they're studying is our mitochondria, organelles in our cells that produce energy. Referring to mitochondria, one scientist noted, "Perhaps no other structure in the cell is so intimately connected to the energy of youth and the decline of the old."

Damage to our mitochondrial DNA is an important factor in aging. As we age, our mitochondria still work, but they've accumulated defects that compromise their symbiotic relationship with the rest of the cell. For one thing, older, defective mitochondria are more prone to rupture, causing them to leak their DNA and other molecules into the cell. The cell then mistakes these bits as bacterial invaders, triggering inflammation. Our neurons are particularly prone to aging mitochondria, which may be one of the reasons our cognitive abilities decline. Unfortunately, scientists have yet to determine the precise sources of mitochondrial damage.

Another contribution to the aging process is the shortening of our telomeres, the protective caps at the ends of our chromosomes. Each time our chromosomes replicate, they lose a bit of these structures. When enough of the telomere is lost, it can no longer divide and replenish itself. Cells that can no longer divide effectively lead to a decline in tissue function, contributing to age-related diseases and decreased lifespan. Telomere shortening in our stem cells is a particular problem: our bodies use stem cells to replenish skin, blood and other tissues. To make matters worse, stress accelerates telomere shortening. That's because the stress hormone, cortisol, further diminishes our telomeres.

Our DNA changes and deteriorates during the normal course of living—which may include exposure to nasty chemicals or radiation. We do have DNA repair mechanisms, but scientists don't know whether the repair mechanisms of exceptionally long-lived people are unusually efficient. As damage to our DNA accumulates and our telomeres shorten, we produce senescent (deteriorating) cells in places where they don't serve any purpose. (When we're injured, however, senescent cells do serve a purpose: they set off inflammation that promotes wound healing and tissue regeneration.) But the ability of our aging bodies to clear senescent cells declines at a faster rate than our immune systems can handle, a situation that leads to chronic, widespread inflammation.

Chronic inflammation, which increases as you age, can also begin with an infection or injury, then morph into a lingering state in which the immune system starts attacking healthy tissue. Chronic inflammation is also linked to stress, smoking, and a declining level of physical activity. Doctors can usually detect chronic inflammation through blood tests that measure specific chemicals released by your immune system.

Our brains also show clear signs of aging: they shrink away from our skulls, leaving a gap. The average 90-year-old has only half of the axons (transmission lines in nerve cells) that he or she once had. In fact, our brains started shrinking at around age 20, when cells start dying faster than they can be replaced, and the axons connecting neurons start to decline. In addition to brain shrinkage, our axons lose their protective insulation (myelin), which further contributes to deterioration.

Interestingly, new research has discovered a plausible reason for the fact that women's brains age more slowly than men's. It has to do with that protective axon insulation, myelin. As you may know, females have two X chromosomes and males have one X and one Y chromosome. In female fetuses, one of the X chromosomes shuts down early in the mother's pregnancy. Its genes go nearly silent. When scientists studied the hippocampi of aging mice, they were astounded to find that the genes in the formerly "silent" X chromosomes had awakened, including the gene that initiates the development of that protective insulation in women's nerve cells.

Dr. Brian Kennedy is the director of the Center for Healthy Longevity at the National University of Singapore, where his research focuses on the biology of aging. He's concluded that healthy aging is about maintaining homeostasis—the "responsive network" in your body that keeps you in equilibrium. "Your body knows how to function in a healthy way," he says. Thus, how well you age depends on how your body responds to the events that happen in the aging process. "We're trying to get to the best state we can be in for the damaged state we're in." Our responsive network, he maintains, is highly malleable and can be influenced by interventions, such as exercise, and, perhaps, some drugs. Most important are interventions that reduce chronic inflammation, a condition that may respond to certain drugs that he's studying in his lab.

Tad Friend, reporting in *The New Yorker* ("Live Long and Prosper") writes, "The body seems to require a Goldilocks solution for pretty much everything....Almost nothing the body does is always bad or always good: we walk a narrow footbridge between atrophy (cells failing to replicate properly) and cancer (cells replicating too well)....And yet, to realize significant gains in longevity, we'll need to significantly disrupt our natural functions."

One influential scientist proposed the "free-radical theory of aging," which is a complicated theory having to do with the accumulation of free radical damage over time. (A free radical is any atom or molecule that has a single unpaired electron in an outer shell.) This theory is controversial, although scientists agree that it has been useful in fostering research. Free radicals come from environmental sources, such as air pollution and ultraviolet rays. Your body also produces free radicals naturally in response to stress and inflammation. When you have too many free radicals gobbling up electrons from stable molecules, it's called oxidative stress. When that happens, cells become damaged and even die.

The free radical theory started the popular movement to consume antioxidants to combat cellular damage. Foods such as blueberries, kale, and dark chocolate—as well as a variety of supplements—are among those believed to combat free radical damage. To test the effects of antioxidants on mortality, scientists conducted 68 clinical trials that included 230,000 participants. The results showed that the supplements did not reduce mortality. In fact, some of the supplements—vitamin A, vitamin E, beta-carotene—actually increased mortality. After conducting a systematic review of studies on antioxidants, the *Therapeutics Journal* concluded that antioxidant supplements "do not promote longevity and do not prevent major cardiovascular events. Therefore, in our view, the prevalent scientific evidence at this moment is that antioxidant supplementation is not a good practice, at least as advice to the general population." You may be trying to lessen free radical damage by eating blueberries and kale. These are good foods, but they aren't going to fix your worn-out mitochondria.

Consumers spend $62 billion a year on "anti-aging" treatments, none of which can reverse the aging process. For now, experts can only recommend exercise and good nutrition. I can definitely get behind the importance of exercise, but I tend to question the "authorities" on the topic of nutrition. In fact, I ignore nutrition studies, especially when they demonize red meat and saturated fat. The information is not trustworthy. The problem is that there are multiple ways to analyze data. Researchers are often looking for results that are publishable. For this reason, they can easily make decisions—consciously or subconsciously—to get the results they want.

A group of researchers called "methodologists" at McMaster University in Canada and Stanford University reviewed 15 studies that were trying to determine whether the consumption of red meat is associated with premature death. They identified 70 different analytical strategies and 1,208 possible combinations of analytic choices. Using sophisticated mathematical techniques, they then determined how the analytical techniques chosen by the researchers might influence the results. Depending on the choices made, the results showed wildly different outcomes: 435 concluded that red meat consumption is associated with an increased risk of premature death; 773 led to the opposite conclusion: the more red meat consumed, the longer people lived. Super ager Warren Buffet's diet is heavy on Mc-Donald's breakfasts, including bacon, egg and cheese biscuits. He dislikes vegetables. His meals often consist of hamburgers, hot dogs, strawberry milkshakes, and cherry Cokes. As he says, "If I eat 2700 calories a day, a quarter of that is Coca-Cola. I drink at least five 12-ounce servings. I do it every day." In fact, Buffett has said that his indulgent diet has been key to his happiness and long lifespan.

Frailty is one measurement of the aging process and is a predictor of adverse health outcomes. According to an article in *The New England Journal of Medicine*, "Frailty is a clinically identifiable state of diminished physiological reserve and increased vulnerability to a broad range of adverse health outcomes." Characteristics include exhaustion (first manifestation), weakness, slowness, physical inactivity, and weight loss (last manifestation). One test of frailty is gait speed: if you walk less than a yard per second, you'll be in the frail category. (In a study of men aged 85 and older, only a quarter of the slowest walkers survived five years, while nearly all the fastest walkers did.) If you don't have any of the frailty characteristics, you're considered "robust." If you exhibit just one or two of these characteristics, you're "pre-frail." I'm happy to report that I may be edging toward "pre-frail," but my weight puts me more in the "robust" camp.

Clinicians may use frailty to determine "risk of death or admission to an institution." In addition, because frailty makes old people more vulnerable to negative outcomes following treatment, clinicians sometimes screen for frailty to help them predict age-related health conditions and to design treatments for building robustness and resilience. In an exhaustive study of various interventions, including exercise, medications, supplements, and nutrition, researchers found that the one intervention that improved people's frailty score was—you guessed it—exercise.

All causes of aging are interconnected, and the accumulated defects in our cellular machinery eventually lead to aging symptoms such as arthritis, fatigue, weakness, and decreased cognition. It all adds up to bodies that simply don't work as well as they did in our youth.

Chapter Seven

Exercise

Even though some super agers and centenarians are not exercisers, most gerontology experts think exercise is important for staying healthy into old age. So do I. I can't remember exactly when I started routinely exercising, but I do recall taking up jogging and aerobic dancing when we lived in Michigan, so it's probably been about 50 years. I didn't keep up with jogging (didn't like it), but I continued with aerobic dancing. My husband and I also played tennis until 1989, at which time the Loma Prieta earthquake destroyed our local courts here in California. Also, my knees gave out.

Euan Ashley, a professor of cardiovascular medicine, genetics, and data science at Stanford, says "Exercise is just the single most important intervention you can think of for your health." In analyzing data of more than half a million people over the course of ten years, he found that exercise reduces our chances of having atrial fibrillation, diabetes, hip fractures, and colon cancer by at least 50 percent. Unlike other interventions that might target one aspect of health, exercise affects nearly every system in your body.

According to neuroscientist Justin Rhodes, exercise can reverse the effects of a genetic bad hand by lowering the risk of a variety of ailments, including heart disease. Exercise also slows aging in several ways: by promoting the growth of stem cells in muscle, expressing genes linked to longevity, and lengthening telomeres. Rhodes contends that we can introduce exercise at any point in our lives and that, for every hour we exercise, we tack two hours onto our life span.

I read in a recent *JAMA* article (2025) that "individuals with the highest levels of physical activity at midlife and late life had 41% and 45% lower risk of all-cause dementia, respectively, compared with those with the lowest levels of physical activity." The study used data collected since 1971 from 5,124 participants.

One of the most important benefits of exercise is reducing inflammation. Sedentary people tend to have higher levels of inflammation than those who exercise regularly. When sedentary people start moving consistently, their inflammation levels generally decline. Apparently, moderate exercise tamps down the release of inflammatory chemicals while at the same time ramping up the release of chemicals that fight inflammation. Exercise can also lower inflammation indirectly. For example, it can lower stress and improve sleep quality.

Exercise also affects fat cells. Certain kinds of fat cells release chemicals into the blood that cause low-grade inflammation. Consistent exercise not only shrinks fat tissue, but, as studies have suggested, physical activity might cause fat cells to produce fewer inflammatory substances. One study showed that a single, moderate, 20-minute treadmill workout sparked a temporary anti-inflammatory response. Of course, to get results, you must make exercise a habit.

Strength is a critical component of how well we'll live as we age. In addition to maintaining overall health, strong muscles protect our joints, improve our balance, and enhance our ability to perform daily activities, from carrying groceries to getting out of a chair. What's more, maintaining muscle strength can significantly reduce the risk of death from all causes.

Muscle degenerates with age. In fact, it begins to decline as early as our 30s. An 80-year-old man will have about 40 percent less muscle tissue than he did at 25. We lose muscle *strength* about two to three times more quickly than we lose muscle *mass*. Our muscle mass, as well as our levels of physical activity, decline steeply after about age 65. After age 75, the decline is even steeper. By age 80 the average person will have lost about eighteen pounds of muscle from his or her peak. But people who maintain higher levels of activity lose much less muscle—more like four to six pounds on average. You can lose muscle scarily fast: a study of twelve healthy volunteers with an average age of 67 who'd stayed in bed for just ten days lost an average of 3.3 pounds of lean muscle mass.

According to Charles Rice, at the University of Western Ontario's Neuromuscular Lab, muscle degeneration involves the nerves that stimulate individual muscle cells to contract. As we age, these nerves start to die. If the muscle is hearing nothing from the nerves, the muscle cell stops contracting, and, eventually it dies too. When we exercise a muscle, we retain those nerves that plug into them.

Even our toes need to be strengthened! Dr. Courtney Conley, who specializes in foot and gait mechanics, says "Toe weakness is the single biggest predictor of falls when we get older." Strong toe flexion (gripping the floor) is crucial in maintaining balance. Poor toe flexor strength increases the risk of falls. If toe strength is compromised, everything up the chain is more vulnerable—ankle, knee, hip, and spine.

A recent study, reported in *JAMA Network Open* (February 13, 2026), showed that muscle strength is associated with lower mortality. Researchers tested the grip strength and lower body strength of 5,472 women aged 63 to 99 years. (Grip strength, which reflects upper body strength, was measured using a hand-held dynamometer; lower body strength was measured using the sit-to-stand test—sitting and rising from a chair five times without using hands.) What I found interesting was the fact that "Muscle strength was associated with lower mortality even in women not meeting the guideline-recommended activity levels" (less than 150 minutes of physical activity per week). In other words, women whose cardiorespiratory fitness was sub-par, but who tested well on strength tests, nevertheless fell into the lower mortality camp. This means that, even if you're disabled and/or use a walker, you can improve your odds for a longer life.

In addition to strength training, we need to do aerobic exercises, such as walking, cycling, and swimming to maintain cardiovascular fitness. Aerobic exercise uses our large muscle groups and increases our heart rates as well as the amount of oxygen our bodies use. By breathing faster and more deeply, we maximize the amount of oxygen in our blood. Our hearts will beat faster, increasing blood flow to our muscles and back to our lungs. Our small blood vessels (capillaries) will widen to deliver more oxygen to our muscles and carry away waste products, such as carbon dioxide and lactic acid. Moreover, aerobic efficiency—our body's capacity to efficiently use oxygen—is deeply tied to the health of our mitochondria, those cellular "engines" responsible for producing energy.

If you want to get technical, you can get your VO_2 max measured. (I've not done this.) VO_2 max is the maximum rate of oxygen consumption attainable during physical exertion. ("V" is for volume, "O_2" for oxygen, and "max" is for maximum.) Because it combines measurements of heart, lung, and muscle efficiency, your VO_2 max is a good measure of your physical capability. The test is unpleasant. You ride an exercise bike or run on a treadmill while wearing a mask. The test measures oxygen consumption and CO_2 production. The peak amount of oxygen you consume—typically close to the point where you can't keep going—yields your VO_2 max. The higher your VO_2 max, the better your cardiovascular and overall physical fitness. For 80-year-old women, a score of less than 15 is low; above average is 20-22; and "elite" is around 30. (For men of the same age, the scores are three to six points higher in each range.)

Your VO_2 max will decline by roughly 10 percent per decade, and then up to 15 percent per decade after the age 50. Once VO_2 max drops below a certain level (typically about 18 ml/kg/min in men and 15 in women), it begins to threaten your ability to live on your own.

Conventional wisdom suggests that it's possible to improve our aerobic capacity by about 13 percent over eight to ten weeks of training, and by 17 percent after 24 to 52 weeks. A small study of nine octogenarian cross-country skiers found that their average VO_2 max was 38 compared to 21 for a control group of untrained octogenarian men, a difference of more than 80 percent. Another study found that boosting elderly subjects' VO_2 max by about 25 percent was equivalent to subtracting twelve years from their age. Of course, that takes a lot of work, especially the cross-country skiing part.

Exercise also helps protect us against age-related cognitive decline. Scientists have found that putting seniors on an aerobic exercise program resulted in a continual expansion of the hippocampus, the part of our brain that is responsible for memory and learning. Researchers found that, when a group of seniors were put on an aerobic exercise program and measured their hippocampal growth at six and twelve months, they found increased growth at each measurement.

Aerobic exercise also re-insulates the transmission lines (axons) that connect brain cells, an improvement that boosts processing speed and makes the connections more reliable. (At around age 40, our neurons start losing their insulation.)

Another study, reported in *JAMA Network Open* (2025), sought to "evaluate the potential critical periods for physical activity in association with dementia risk." To do this, a team of scientists studied the exercise habits of nearly 2,000 people ages 54 to 71 and older, using data collected from 1979 to 2023 in the Framingham Heart Study. Their conclusion: "...individuals with the highest levels of physical activity at midlife and late life had 41% and 45% lower risk of all-cause dementia, respectively, compared with those with the lowest levels of physical activity, a statistically significant difference."

Researchers have long known that one beneficial intervention for patients with heart disease is "cardiac rehabilitation" (aka exercise). Cardiac rehabilitation is a medically supervised program for people who have had a heart attack, heart failure, angioplasty or heart surgery. The program has been proven to reduce heart attacks, hospitalization, and cardiovascular deaths. But the programs are perennially underused. Only about one-quarter of eligible patients participate. This is especially true for people in their 70s and 80s. Getting to the exercise facility may be a problem, but the biggest hindrance is fear of falling and worry that the activity might be harmful.

For my own exercise routine, I use the online Jazzercise On Demand program. It costs about $25.00 a month. Before Covid, I participated in an in-person Jazzercise class, but it shut down during the pandemic. By the time the class started again, I felt like I was too old, which is why I opted for the online version. I recommend it. The Jazzercise catalog offers plenty of options, letting you choose routines that work best for you. You could also consider SilverSneakers, an exercise program geared to older people. It offers both in-person and online classes and is free if you're over 65 and participate in one of the "select Medicare plans."

My workout consists of a 20- to 30-minute Jazzercize "dance cardio" routine, followed by a 10-minute upper-body strength routine, using five-pound weights. After those exercises, I do a series of yoga stretches. I follow this routine religiously every Monday, Wednesday, and Saturday mornings, although I'd rather sit. On Tuesdays, I attend a weekly yoga class that focuses on strength, flexibility, and balance. The class isn't easy and requires getting down and up from the floor. I get additional exercise in my weekly routines of golf on Thursdays, housecleaning on Fridays, and yardwork on Sundays. Did I mention that I'm addicted to routines?

In their efforts to maintain strength and health, most of the old people I know make it a habit to go for walks on most days. It's great exercise. But the older we get, our walking techniques may start getting sloppy, which causes us to underuse some muscles and overuse some joints. At worst, we might sway from side to side like a penguin or even shuffle. (I catch myself walking like a penguin sometimes when my hips hurt.) Typically, many—if not most—people's walking techniques consist of a series of forward falls blocked abruptly by the forward leg, a style that jams our hips and every other weight-bearing joint. At the same time, our butt and leg muscles are underused. You're supposed to engage your butt muscles when you walk. As Esther Gokhale, the posture lady, writes, "The buttock and leg muscles contract strongly to propel the body forward, thus getting the exercise they need while the back is spared unnecessary wear and tear." I've found that it's hard to think about contracting my butt muscles to propel me forward. But what's easier to remember is keeping my back leg straight and the heel on the ground. When you do that, your glute muscles engage.

My weekly golfing is pretty much the only time I do any serious walking. Our house is at the end of a steep mountain road, which makes walking in my neighborhood too strenuous. My husband and I belong to the Monterey Bay Seniors Golf Association, a group of great guys whose company I enjoy. (Only two of us players are women.) I'm a terrible golfer, but nobody seems to mind.

I've always assumed that golfing was good for us. To confirm this assumption, I recently discovered that researchers have studied the benefits of golf for old people. The University of Southern California has an Institute for Therapeutic Golf Science. Their studies have found that "in as few as 10 weeks, participation in the sport—which gets players striding up and down inclines and squatting to place and recover balls—increases walking ability and balance, improves performance on cognitive and memory tests, and reduces blood markers for inflammation." The Institute also stresses the importance of the social aspects of golf. I don't know how much longer we can continue with this sport, but for now it's great exercise and gets us outdoors.

I don't want to give the impression that I easily sail through my muscle- and energy-demanding routines. I do get sore and tired—with some activities more than others. And, of course, each year they get harder. But I'm persuaded that the benefits are real, so I will soldier on.

I asked four friends to tell me about their exercise routines. Susan, born in 1933, has congestive heart failure and severe osteoporosis. She's had breast cancer, the treatment for which was a mastectomy, chemotherapy and radiation, followed by breast reconstruction. She's shattered her upper leg bone in three places, and has also broken her pelvis, nose, wrist, jaw and ribs. She's had both knees replaced as well as both shoulders. The surgery on her right shoulder left her with no rotator cuff. (This is tough: the rotator cuff is a group of muscles and tendons around the shoulder joint that connects the shoulder blade to the upper arm bone. It plays a crucial role in stabilizing the shoulder, elevating and rotating the arm, and ensuring the head of the humerus stays securely placed in the shoulder socket.) She's had three spinal fusion surgeries on her neck and lower back—six fusions in all. (Spinal fusion surgeries connect one or more vertebrae together either by bone grafting, using an artificial bone substitute, and/or adding hardware such as screws or plates.)

Nevertheless, Susan is functioning very well, a fact her cardiologist attributes to her exercise routine—one that makes me tired just thinking about. She does at least 150 minutes of strenuous aerobic exercise a week—usually at least 30 minutes a day. She uses both a bike and a treadmill. On the bike, she keeps her heart rate at 80 percent of maximum for her age, frequently pushing herself extra hard for brief periods. On the treadmill, she either keeps her heart rate elevated throughout 30 minutes or raises it in spurts by doing extra-strenuous intervals. On days when she "just can't face the machines" she walks at least 2.5 miles at a pace that keeps her heart rate elevated. In addition to the aerobic workout, two to three times a week she performs a variety of routines using heavy-duty elastic bands and weights to strengthen her arms, shoulders, legs and hips. She also does lots of lunges and squats. Whew!

Donna, born in 1927, is a walker—but she doesn't *use* a walker. In her younger days, she walked over 5,000 miles in three walks for peace in the U.S. and Russia. The first, when she was 59, took her from Los Angeles to Washington, DC. The next year, she walked and bused from Leningrad to Moscow. In 1988, she participated in The American-Soviet Peace Walk from Washington, DC, to San Francisco. Now, she says, "I walk at every opportunity."

Donna lives in a retirement community where she walks its one-mile perimeter several times a week. She also walks a third of a mile to the dining room and a quarter mile to the health services office where she takes a variety of pills, some of which are for heart health. (She's had one of the valves in her heart replaced and has a pacemaker—a small, surgically implanted, battery-powered device used to regulate heart rhythm and rate.) In addition to her walks around her community, Donna regularly uses the community pool for an hour of water-walking—resistance training that provides a good cardiovascular workout.

Before getting out of bed in the morning, Donna spends about ten minutes doing stretches—"nothing grand or impressive, but I feel more flexible and spry when I roll out and stand up." Not only is Donna spry, she's an inveterate community organizer, as exemplified by the Pacemakers Club she started "so we can meet for lunch once a month and tell our stories and laugh a lot."

Michelle, born in 1936, became significantly disabled in 2019. Her spinal column collapsed, damaging her spinal cord at two places in her neck (C4 and C5). Standing and walking were difficult and painful. "For a long time" she says, "I needed someone to cook for me because I couldn't grocery shop and I couldn't stand in the kitchen for any length of time." To walk, she needed either a walker or two walking sticks. "After lots of physical therapy and working out at home, I'm now quite independent. I consider myself within the normal range."

The key to Michelle's recovery has been physical therapy, a practice she continues to this day. She stresses the importance of evaluating physical therapists to ensure you get a good one, then "follow their directions and continue to practice the exercises that you learn." She also performs Pilates exercises and uses a stationary bike, watching TV as she pedals. To ensure consistency in following a routine, Michelle meets with a friend by phone every morning. They exercise together for 45 minutes.

"When I became disabled," Michelle says, "I had no interest in walking. However, my neighbor needed a companion for her dog, Sophie, during the day. For the next five years, Sophie walked herself over to my house, pushed open the front door, and came in. We always went for walks twice a day."

It's clear that Michelle is not one to "go it alone." Fundamental to her successful recovery have been three helpers: a physical therapist, a friend, and a dog.

George, born in 1935, is an actor. Some years ago, we watched him in a role that required him to squat. No problem for him, although he was probably about 80 at that time. I was impressed. My knees wouldn't allow me to do that. For this book, I asked him about his exercise routine, which he performs most days, and which makes my routine look meager in comparison. I won't list each routine, but here's how he says it starts: "Stretch hands to sky, then to toes; stretch hands forward, then back to sky, then horizontally." He does these moves 100 times while rocking back and forth from his toes to heels. His exercise routine lasts an hour and also includes 25 push-ups; 100 sit-ups; a variety of moves with eight-pound weights; 100 reps of bicycle pumps while lying on his back; a variety of moves using a resistance band; holding the plank pose for 50 counts, as well as holding that pose while alternately bending one knee towards his ear—50 reps on each leg. (The plank pose is done on the floor, using your hands or elbows to raise your upper body and your flexed toes to raise your lower body, keeping the length of your body rigidly straight and off the floor.) He also does a variety of other yoga poses, including tree pose, which requires balancing on one foot.

George is motivated, he says, by the idea that he's "training" for the annual Sacred Peace Walk, an interfaith journey of 60 miles from Las Vegas to the Nevada Nuclear Test Site. He's participated in this walk for 15 years. Is there a correlation between peace walks and a long life?

You probably know people who have lived into their nineties without regularly engaging in activities that demand strength and stamina. Perhaps they're even couch potatoes. Still, given the plethora of studies proving the benefits of exercise for health and longevity, I think we stand a better chance of beating the odds against frailty and debilitation by getting off the couch.

Chapter Eight

The longevity industry

Scientists don't fully understand why our lifespans are naturally limited, but they're trying to get to the bottom of it. There's money to be made. In fact, the longevity market is rapidly growing into a multibillion-dollar industry fueled by an influx of funding from investors, academic institutions, biotech leaders, and entrepreneurs. In 2023, the industry generated $65 billion in revenue and is projected to reach $314 billion by 2030.

The market includes complementary and alternative medicines, gene sequencing, and anti-aging therapies and products. Part of this effort includes the study of *biomarkers*—indicators that measure inflammation, hormone levels, patterns of gene expression, and other aging markers. For example, the BRCA gene is a biomarker for predicting breast cancer; various enzymes and proteins are biomarkers that may indicate heart disease.

Using this new information, an increasing number of industries are devoting their resources to search for anti-aging treatments. In fact, more than 700 biotech companies are focused on aging and longevity. One such company is Altos Labs, based in San Diego, California. Their website states, "Our mission is to reverse disease, injury and the disabilities that occur throughout life by restoring cell health and resilience through cell rejuvenation." In typical tech-company-speak, the site explains that they are "developing multi-scale generative models to unravel the language of cell health, organ health and the complex relationship between them, across biological hierarchies." Their plan is to reprogram cells, or, as they describe it, to "push the reset button."

Altos Labs is beginning this effort by growing the skin cells of middle-aged people in petri dishes and flicking on "special genetic switches." That is, the scientists reprogram the cells to erase the properties associated with age. In examining the cells they've altered, the researchers found them to be 25 and 30 biological years younger than they had been at the start of the experiment. Altos Labs isn't the only company experimenting on cells. Apparently, the science of resetting cells has taken off, with researchers hoping that their work will result in a tool, as Altos Labs says, that "could heal an aging body at the molecular level, regardless of the disease."

The longevity industry includes businesses which, for a price, offer programs and products to help you live a longer, healthier life. For example, Equinox, a health club of sorts, offers "the definitive approach to full health optimization." For $40,000 a year, you get biometric analysis, a sleep coach who will conduct two private half-hour sessions a month, a twice-monthly nutrition coach, and a thrice-weekly personal trainer. Fountain Life, another longevity clinic, offers a semi-annual Platinum Trip where, for $70,000, you can meet with longevity scientists, invest in their experimental therapies, and get some of their new therapies for your own use.

Peter Attia, author of *Outlive: The Science and Art of Longevity*, offers advice, programs, and products to help you live a longer, healthier life. He's an MD, with a medical degree from Stanford University School of Medicine. He also trained for five years at the Johns Hopkins Hospital in general surgery and spent two years at the National Institutes of

Health as a surgical oncology fellow with the National Cancer Institute. As a medical practitioner, Attia became disenchanted with what he calls "Medicine 2.0"— "reactive" medicine that focuses on treatment rather than prevention. He calls his program "Medicine 3.0."—medicine that's centered on "early intervention, prevention, and understanding individual risk factors long before they manifest as disease." Medicine 3.0 focuses on "lifestyle optimization," including exercise, nutrition, sleep, and what he calls "exogenous molecules" (drugs, hormones, or supplements).

You can participate in Medicine 3.0 by joining his Biograph program, "The world's most advanced preventive health clinic," where you learn your risk factors for cardiovascular disease, cancer, or Alzheimer's based on your genetics, family history, and biomarkers. After that, you're prescribed "targeted actions to mitigate those risks decades before the first symptoms appear." The program includes over 20 evaluations, including a six-hour initial testing visit, the results of which lead to personalized health insights and risk assessments as well as an analysis of over 1,000 data points (bio-markers). If you sign up for the $15,000 per year "Black" membership, you'll receive expert guidance from the organization's nutrition and exercise consultants, as well as ongoing monitoring.

I have mixed feelings about Dr. Attia's efforts. On the one hand, I think his notion of preventive care is sensible and I admire his expertise. But his program is unaffordable for most people. (A course on longevity costs $2,500.) Plus, now there's the sleaze factor: Attia's name pops up more than 1,700 times in the Epstein files. Apparently, Attia was fascinated by Epstein's wealth and access to influential people—qualities that can help researchers push their careers to the next level. Of course, now Attia is sorry for his relationship with Epstein.

Even if I disregard costs and sleazy relationships, I'm not sure I'd want all that biometric information about myself or to spend the rest of my life "actively working to prevent the conditions that have plagued previous generations." I must admit, however, that I have some biometric information on file with 23andMe. In searching my records on their site I was relieved to discover that I don't have the gene (APOE) that increases the risk of Alzheimer's disease.

You may have heard of Bryan Johnson, who spends about $2 million a year on treatments to boost his health and prolong his life. In a Netflix documentary called "Don't Die," Johnson—born in 1977—shows us the ways he has turned his home into a lab. Watching the documentary, it appears that he spends most of his days on his health regimen. His objective, as he describes it, is to "maximally slow the speed of my biological aging. My goal: one year of chronological time passes and my biological age stays the same." In fact, he says that his health regimen has reversed his biological age 5.1 years. (Studies have refuted this.) His previous career as a venture capitalist and tech entrepreneur provides the funds for his longevity endeavors. (One of his companies was acquired by PayPal for $800 million in 2013.)

Johnson's health regimen strikes me as extreme. For example, he eats breakfast, lunch, and dinner before noon each day: breakfast at 6:45 AM (protein powder, nuts, blueberries, collagen protein, coca, and extra virgin olive oil); lunch at 9:00 AM (black lentils, broccoli, garlic, mushrooms, hemp seeds, fermented foods); dinner at 11:00 AM (sweet potato, avocado, tomatoes, chickpeas, radishes, chili powder). He takes over 100 pills each day, which include supplements and prescription drugs. His company, Blueprint, sells the supplements. For example, for $49, you can buy his "longevity mix." (Some people who consumed this mix complained that it was making them sick.)

His day is filled with a variety of routines, such as his 60- to 90-minute daily workout sessions that focus on cardiovascular exercises, strength, flexibility, and balance. His skin regimen includes cleansers, moisturizers, and serums as well as the use of a protective umbrella that he carries outside to protect his skin. He washes his hair with a "scalp-stimulating shampoo," massaging his scalp with a soft silicone brush. He also applies a serum to his scalp. For six minutes a day he wears a red-light therapy cap to promote hair growth. In the morning and night, he brushes his teeth with fluoride-free toothpaste, flosses, scrapes his tongue, uses a Waterpik, and follows up with mouthwash. At night he wears a device to combat teeth grinding while sleeping.

Speaking of sleep, Johnson reports, "I achieved the best recorded sleep score in history. Eight months of perfect, 100% sleep." A few of the things he does to achieve this record include a 30- to 60-minute wind-down routine, taking 300 micrograms of melatonin, dimming the lights one to two hours before bed (and switching to red light), and sleeping on a temperature-controlled mattress. One last thing: he measures his nighttime erections and claims his score is equal to an 18-year-old, thanks to this protocol. (Doesn't that interrupt his sleep?) Maybe it's just me, but I think he's kind of creepy. If you want to learn more and buy his products, you can visit his website, Blueprint.

Two drugs, rapamycin and metformin, keep popping up in discussions about longevity as well as in the practices of some of the gurus. Both Peter Attia and Bryan Johnson, for example, take these drugs. Rapamycin is an antibiotic originally discovered in the soil of Easter Island. Prior to 2009, it was primarily used as an immune suppressor for people receiving organ transplants to prevent them from rejecting the foreign organ. Though rapamycin is an immunosuppressive drug, researchers, experimenting with mice, have found that it can enhance immune function and reduce inflammation. They surmise that optimal health calls for a fine balance between excessive inflammation and heightened susceptibility to infection. As Dr.

Ramakrishnan, author of *Why We Die*, notes, "It may well be that low or intermittent doses of rapamycin…can confer most of their benefits without serious risks. But we need long-term studies on their safety and efficacy before they can be used to target aging in humans." (I heard, in an interview with Dr. Attia on the "60 Minutes" news program, that he has quit taking the drug because he developed sores in his mouth.)

Metformin is the most widely prescribed drug for people with type 2 diabetes. It reduces blood sugar. Researchers found that diabetics on metformin lived longer than diabetics on other drugs and that they also lived longer than nondiabetics—although this research is now being questioned. As with rapamycin, metformin has shown to slow down the aging process in laboratory animals. In humans, preliminary studies suggest that metformin may slow the aging process and increase life expectancy by improving the body's responsiveness to insulin, as well as by acting as an antioxidant and improving blood vessel health. Despite its widespread use, the mechanisms that cause metformin's favorable effects on aging are largely unknown. Further, not all individuals who are prescribed metformin derive the same benefit, and some develop side effects. As *Harvard Health Publishing* reports, "While the research so far is promising, we need more compelling evidence before endorsing its widespread use for people without diabetes. But, for clinical researchers hoping to repurpose an old medicine as a new wonder drug, metformin would seem like a great place to start."

N.A.D.+ is another supplement that longevity seekers are taking. (N.A .D.+ stands for nicotinamide adenine dinucleotide.) It's a molecule found in all cells that's essential for repairing damage and encouraging healing. Because this molecule decreases with age, some researchers think that elevating it in our bodies through infusions or supplements could slow the aging process. For hundreds of dollars per session, you can go to a longevity clinic to get weekly or biweekly IV infusions of N.A.D.+. Or you can buy pills, starting at about $20.00 a month. Because such treatments are marketed as dietary supplements or wellness products, they don't require approval by the Food and Drug Administration. For now, scientists don't know whether this therapy improves our health span or life span. For one thing, they don't know whether the decline in N.A.D.+ does, in fact, speed the aging process or if it's just associated with it. Evidence is scarce. As Dr. Eduardo Chini, who runs a metabolic research lab at the Mayo Clinic in Jacksonville, Florida, says, "I don't think you can say there is or there isn't evidence that N.A.D.+ drives the aging process."

Some researchers and anti-aging influencers believe that exchanging the plasma in your blood with a donor's plasma or with a special substitute fluid helps to slow aging. They argue that the treatment removes the inflammatory antibodies and proteins that may drive biological aging. The treatment requires that you get hooked up to a machine that draws out your blood, separates and discards the plasma portion, replaces it with donor plasma or other fluid, then returns your blood. A small study of 42 participants, with an average age of 65, found that the blood of those who got plasma exchange therapy had lower concentrations of the biological compounds that accumulate with age than did the blood of a control group.

Of course, many scientists are skeptical, arguing that the anti-aging benefits of plasma exchange for healthy people have never been proven in large clinical trials. Moreover, the studies haven't shown how long its effects last or proven that the treatment will help people live longer or healthier. One trial of 350 Alzheimer's patients who underwent plasma therapy over about 14 months saw slower cognitive decline than those who received a placebo treatment. If you want to try it, count on spending thousands of dollars a session at one of the longevity clinics that offers it.

Another practice recommended by longevity gurus is intermittent fasting—diet regimens that include repeated periods of zero or very low-calorie intake. The most common fasting protocols are these:

- Time-restricted eating—consuming all food in a 4- to 12-hour window

- Alternate-day fasting—either abstaining from food every other day or eating no more than 500 calories on that day

- Limiting meals to 500 calories on two days per week

Mark Mattson, at the Johns Hopkins School of Medicine, has been studying fasting for 30 years. He argues that, because ancient hunter-gatherer humans went for long periods without food, we have evolved to benefit from taking breaks from eating. Here's the benefit: after your cells have used up all the glucose available from either the last meal you ate, or from the glycogen stored in your liver and muscles—a period that's typically about 12 hours after your last meal—your body enters a fasted state in which stored fat is converted to ketone bodies. (Ketones are acids your body makes when it's using fat instead of glucose as an alternative energy source.) Mattson and others believe that the shift between sources of energy, called metabolic switching, triggers key adaptive stress responses, including increased DNA repair and the breakdown and recycling of defective cellular components.

A *PubMed* article notes that intermittent fasting has "the potential to prevent and treat disease, but the effect on cellular aging and the molecular mechanisms involved are only beginning to be unraveled." Nevertheless, the article states, "In humans, the alternation of fasting and refeeding periods is accompanied by positive effects on risk factors for aging, diabetes, autoimmunity, cardiovascular disease, neurodegeneration and cancer."

Even though I've been aware of intermittent fasting as a health-promoting regimen, I've never been interested in pursuing this practice, mostly because the idea smacks of deprivation. But now it occurs to me that my husband and I have been practicing intermittent fasting for decades. That is, we practice the time-restricted diet, eating all of our food within a 4- to 12-hour window. We eat dinner at 5:30 PM and breakfast around 7:00 AM. That's more than 12 hours between these meals.

There's no shortage of advice about how to live a longer, healthier life. You may have read about or seen a documentary on "blue zones," those supposedly amazing places—from Okinawa, Japan, to Ikaria, Greece—where a disproportionate number of people live into a very old age. Dr. Saul Newman, a research fellow at the University College London Center for Longitudinal Studies, debunks the blue-zone research with studies of his own. He found undetected errors in every blue zone.

As he notes in an interview, "there's only one data source for human ages, and that's documents." For one thing, he found a lack of documentation certifying people's deaths, including cases where families who had not registered their relatives' deaths were getting their social security money. He discovered many cases of age fraud—people claiming to be older than they were for cultural or financial benefit. For example, in Greece he found that at least 72 percent of centenarians were dead, missing, or essentially pension-fraud cases. In one of the fraud cases, "the world's oldest man" was actually his younger brother. They'd swapped documents. In the United States, Newman found that at least 17 percent of people purported to be over the age of 100 were, in fact, either clerical errors, missing, or dead.

The Blue Zone documentary shows old people in Okinawa happily tending to their gardens. In reality, Okinawans aren't gardeners. The government of Japan has been measuring life in Okinawa and other prefectures since 1975. Their records indicate that, in the matter of growing gardens, Okinawa is third to last after Tokyo and Osaka, where everyone lives in a high-rise. Government records also show that Okinawans are third to last in their consumption of root and leafy green vegetables. In fact, Newman reports that, according to government data Okinawa "lands at the bottom of the health pile."

Loma Linda, California, is purportedly the single U.S. blue zone. It's known for its high concentration of Seventh-day Adventists, who eat a mostly plant-based diet. Newman says the CDC measured Loma Linda for lifespan and found that "…it is completely and utterly unremarkable."

Incidentally, Newman and other researchers question the reliability of the claim that Jean Calment lived to age 122. He says she burned many of her personal papers when she moved into a nursing home, and that demographers trusted the fact that she was well known enough in her town that it would have been hard to fudge her age. Other researchers maintain that Jean's daughter, Yvonne, who was born in 1898, assumed her mother's identity when Jean died of tuberculosis in 1933. This matter is still unsettled.

Years ago, *National Geographic* presented something called "longevity zones," which had the same hallmarks as the blue zones, but in this case the zones were in Soviet Georgia, where yogurt was the secret to a long life; Vilcabamba Valley, in Ecuador; and the Hunza Valley in Pakistan. In every single case the findings were based on what Newman calls "rubbish recordkeeping."

Newman reminds us that the core of science is reproducibility. Not only have the blue zone results not been reproduced, but the underlying blue zone data has never been published. In fact, he writes, "…the science of extreme longevity continues as an immense joke." Nevertheless, Newman recommends behaviors that will increase your lifespan: don't smoke; don't drink alcohol; exercise.

There's also this: the greatest predictor of longevity is the good fortune to be born into a comfortable, well-educated family in a developed country—having enough of the basic necessities such as food, housing, and clean water, as well as adequate income and access to health care. In the U.S., America's richest now live a dozen years longer than its poorest.

I won't be around long enough to learn whether longevity gurus such as Peter Attia and Bryan Johnson will live exceptionally long and healthy lives. It would be interesting to find out. As to embarking on such efforts myself, it's too late. Besides, I'm not willing to focus my remaining days on trying to adjust my biomarkers.

Part Three: Accommodating and Adjusting

Chapter Nine

Living arrangements for old people

Most of us over the age of 65 live in communities of one sort or another, either among the wider community or in retirement communities. We are "aging in place;" that is, we're staying put in our homes. Some of us share homes with unrelated housemates or in cohousing communities. Only about 2 percent (one million) of us live in assisted living facilities, and 4.5 percent (about 1.5 million) of us live in nursing homes, although 35 percent of us will stay in a nursing home at some point in our lives.

My husband and I are aging in place. We live in a small mountain town on California's Central Coast. Our two-story house is at the end of a narrow steep road and is surrounded by redwoods. This living situation can be dangerous when forest fires come near, as happened in the 2020 CZU Lightning Complex fire. We had to evacuate, choosing to go to a family cabin in the Sierras. The day after we left that cabin, the Creek Fire burned it to the ground. Such is life now in California. (We returned home to find our home unscathed).

Wildfires aside, as we approach 90, my husband and I occasionally discuss the idea of living in a retirement community—a place where we can be confident our needs will be met. It's tempting, but we're staying put for now. We built our home here thirty-plus years ago to suit our needs and visions of a "dream home." We are attached to this place.

Surrounded by wildlife, towering trees, and mountains, our home provides us with daily pleasure. Plus, we have a small, five-family neighborhood, the members of which look out for each other, even though no one is close by. (Zoning laws on our road restrict us to ten-acre minimum building sites.) One of our neighbors was five years old when we moved in. We've enjoyed watching him grow, get married and become a father. His grandparents—now deceased—lived in our neighborhood. His mother lives here too. Though we've become slow and creaky, we're managing here with a little help from neighbors and occasional gardeners and handymen.

Living on your own can be risky, as was made clear when, in February of 2025, we learned of the tragic deaths of the actor Gene Hackman and his wife, Betsy Arakawa, who was his primary caregiver. Arakawa, 30 years younger than Hackman, died from complications of hantavirus, leaving him abandoned in their home. Information from Hackman's pacemaker suggests that he remained alive for six days before he died. Because he suffered from Alzheimer's disease, he was unable to care for himself or seek help.

To avoid such a fate, old people who live alone often use devices, such as the wearable emergency buttons that call either 911 or family members. Another strategy is to check in with someone every day. For example, my husband's grandmother called her son's home every morning to let the family know that all was well. My mother raised her window shade every day to let her neighbors know she was all right.

Many of my friends have moved to communities that combine independent living with medical and social support. These living arrangements are called Continuing Care Retirement Communities (CCRCs), of which there are about 2,000 in the U.S. CCRCs offer independent living, assisted living, and skilled nursing, all on the same grounds. Residents can transition between these levels of care as their needs change, without having to move to a different facility. Some CCRCs are located within or near university campuses where residents can take classes, attend athletic and performing arts events, and volunteer as teaching and lab assistants.

The costs of CCRCs vary, depending on the location, floor plan, service plan, and contract type. Most of these communities charge an entry fee. The average initial payment is about $402,000, but the amounts can range widely, from $40,000 to more than two million. After moving in, residents pay monthly maintenance or service fees ranging from $5,000 to $10,000. For example, at Mirabella, a CCRC located on the campus of Arizona University, the entry fees start at $490,600 and monthly fees start at $5,541.

CCRC organizations recommend joining them sooner rather than later. For one thing, you're required to start off by living independently. That is, you can't immediately move to an assisted living or nursing facility. For this reason, CCRCs typically perform a health evaluation on prospective residents as a part of the application process. If you don't meet the health criteria, your application will be denied. Another reason the CCRCs recommend joining earlier is that the move will be easier when you're younger. You'll also have more time to enjoy the variety of activities and exercise programs, take advantage of the meals, and make new friends. Incidentally, at CCRCs, as with other retirement communities, women usually outnumber the men. One of my classmates moved to a facility where the ratio is 70 single men to 240 single women.

Because I have friends who live in CCRCs, I've visited half a dozen or so. They can be very appealing, and my friends have all been satisfied with their new homes. This was not true for my dad. For one year, my parents moved to a beautiful retirement community in Laguna Beach, California. It was my mother's idea. She liked the classes and community gatherings that were offered. But my father felt out of place. He characterized the men in the community as blazer-wearing geezers walking their poodle dogs. After the year was up, they moved back to their small town in the Sierra foothills where my dad was a well-known community leader.

Unlike my father, Janet and Paul are happy with their choice of Pilgrim Place, the retirement community they joined decades ago. Their community, in Southern California, was founded in 1915 as a "missionary home," a place for Congregational Church missionaries to rest and recover between assignments. Now a fully functioning CCRC, its 350 residents can choose from a variety of housing arrangements spread over its 32-acre grounds. Janet and Paul live in a stand-alone cottage on a curved, tree-lined street. In addition to single-family houses, residents may also live in duplex and apartment units. The community's origins are reflected in its social-action focus. As its website says, the community "works together to promote justice, peace and care of the earth."

I asked Janet to describe their lives at Pilgrim Place:

> Our retirement community is a very vibrant institution, full of opportunities to participate in many kinds of activities, all planned by residents. Currently, the major focus includes protests and postcard writing about political issues, identifying institutional priorities for the next five years, and efforts to increase the resident fund for assistance to those whose resources run low. At other times, it may be movement or

theater. Some write and share papers on a variety of topics while others read Emily Dickinson together. Of course, all activities are optional, so we claim down time as well. Resident leadership results in a very active intellectually as well as physically strong community.

Such a lovely place to be creative! I have learned to weave here in a small guild led by volunteer teachers who encourage us, challenge us, and correct us when we get lost. Paul has become an abstract acrylic artist and has sold nearly 100 paintings. I have had vegetable and flower gardens both at our home and in one of the community gardens. We sell excess produce from these gardens weekly.

Our unique noon meal, required of all independent residents, is served buffet style to residents who are randomly assigned seats at tables of six or seven. The result is not only the avoidance of cliques or being left out at the meal but also the development of relationships among the entire community.

Our children are very happy that we live here, even though that means a distance away from most of them. They have confidence in our staff, as do we, and know that we will be cared for even when they cannot be here in person. We have lived independently here for the past 26 years. So far we have been able to participate as we choose and yet be supported when we have a need for assistance.

In a later message to me, Janet mentioned another advantage: "two tech gurus we can schedule to fix things for us." Tempting!

Zeva and Frank, college classmates of mine, recently moved into a CCRC in Marin County, California. Their move was precipitated by struggles with health and home maintenance issues. Before selecting their new home, they visited two other CCRC communities, selecting the one located nearest to their children. It's an eleven-story apartment-style facility with views of San Pablo Bay. As with other CCRCs, their new home offers access to a clinic staffed by nurses and a physician, as well as additional residential options as needed, including assisted living, skilled nursing center, and memory care. As Zeva notes, "These amenities are, in fact, the primary support we sought."

I was impressed to learn that the facility helped with both downsizing and moving, providing up to 12 hours of help with a "designer/organizer" who, Zeva writes, "was extremely helpful, both helping us determine what would fit into our new, smaller unit, and also recommending sources for new furniture that we would need. The movers packed all of our belongings and they and the designer unpacked them, so that when we moved in all our belongings were put away and nicely organized!" The facility also built two new shelving units: "one for our TV and stereo equipment and another for bookshelves. Both were beautifully finished and very professional." Zeva notes that the maintenance people are "very pleasant to work with and always available."

Their spacious, light-filled apartment includes "a well-appointed kitchen with full-size refrigerator/freezer, stovetop, combination microwave/convection oven, sink and plenty of storage and counter space." While Zeva and Frank choose to eat breakfast in their apartment, the community offers three meals a day in three different locations: a dining hall "with stunning views," a cafeteria-style option, and a "pickup area with daily sandwiches, drinks, desserts, etc." You can take food from the latter two options back to your apartment.

Included in their new setting is a business center, fitness center, art room, libraries, auditorium, hair salon, apartment-adjacent laundry room, and a spacious area for large-scale entertaining. They even have a "trash room," where the "staff empties and removes whatever we put there." Outdoor spaces include lawns for putting and croquet, as well as gardens where Zeva takes her daily walk. Shuttle services take residents to "nearby outings, musical and other events, shopping, appointments, etc." Their weekly housekeeper not only cleans their apartment, but also changes their bed, using sheets that are provided by the facility.

"Perhaps the most appealing," Zeva writes,

> ...are the interesting, friendly, supportive helpful fellow residents and staff. Early on, as new members, we were invited to a new residents' dinner where we met many people. We were then invited to join different groups for dinner, meeting even more people. We were assigned a mentor—a fellow resident who gave us a tour and many ideas of available services. We also have a hospitality person, also a fellow resident, who is available to help us, and who is there for us.

As Zeva sums it up, "We feel we have made a choice that is working well for us."

Another housing option for seniors is assisted living. These facilities allow you to remain somewhat independent while, at the same time, providing help with daily activities, such as bathing, dressing, and laundry. Assisted living facilities typically provide 24-hour on-site staff and up to three prepared meals a day, as well as housekeeping, transportation services, and opportunities for social and recreational activities. The facilities range in size from as few as 25 residents to 120. Some offer luxury apartments as well as amenities, such as spas and bars.

The average cost of assisted living in the U.S. is around $5,900 per month, but this can vary significantly based on location, care needs, and the type of community. Factors such as apartment size and care requirements influence the total cost, as do additional services, such as hospice care. Some communities may have all-inclusive pricing, while others use tiered or *a la carte* systems. At the facility I'm familiar with, monthly costs start at $4,775 per month and range up to $8,500, the average being $6,097.

Nick, a retired professor of religion in his mid-nineties, is being treated for end-stage congestive heart failure, a condition that requires careful monitoring and assistance. At one point, his condition necessitated a ten-day hospital stay, after which he was moved to a skilled nursing facility. At that facility, as Nick reported, residents were housed two to a room, where interruptions by staff seemed unending. Even though he'd been seen by occupational and physical therapists, there was "little opportunity to get up and walk." What's more, the facility offered "a lot of rich food."

After consultations with his doctors, it became clear that Nick wasn't strong enough to go home following his stint at the nursing home. For this reason, moving to an assisted living facility made the most sense. Nick now lives at Paradise Assisted Care. As Nick says, "It is easier and less expensive to have me cared for here rather than at home, which would require hired help." The facility looks like a large home, offering 29 single-occupancy rooms. Compared to the skilled nursing facility, Nick says that Paradise is "a saner place with few interruptions and a well-trained staff that provides compassionate care. Requests for assistance are met quickly and efficiently." He calls Paradise a "minimalist service place"—that is, residents must provide their own physical and occupational therapy as well as outings, an arrangement Nick prefers. (If needed, visits by physical and occupational therapists from a specialized agency are easily arranged, as happens automatically following a hospital stay).

Paradise does provide exercise and music programs, and his wife and daughter often take him out for "field trips" and to his frequent medical appointments. He prefers the simple meals offered by Paradise, "with an occasional cookie or scoop of strawberry ice cream, always strawberry!" Nick can easily socialize with others, either by walking to other rooms or joining people in group settings, including the dining room. Given his interactions with other residents and his many visitors, Nick has no shortage of social engagement. He's been assigned to a conversation table, which, he says "has its limitations—conversations focus on Bingo and the number of chocolates a person has won." While he admits that he's exaggerating a bit, he's found that it's up to him to introduce different conversational gambits. Conversational limitations or not, Nick says, "I am pleased with my life in Paradise."

Donna, a former lawyer, cello player, and college classmate of mine, recently moved from her condo, where she'd lived for 20 years, to an assisted living facility near Washington, D.C. Her move was precipitated by problems with her legs. She was unable to stand or walk, although time spent in rehab solved that problem. Nevertheless, returning to her condo—a fourth-floor walk-up—was clearly impractical. Unlike Nick's facility, Donna's new home is a six-story apartment-style complex. Her apartment has the same amount of living space as her condo, and includes a separate bedroom, a mini-kitchen with sink, microwave, and refrigerator, and a balcony with chairs for outside sitting and space to hold her potted plants. The facility provides three meals a day, as well as a wide range of activities that are available from 10:00 in the morning until dinnertime. The activities include discussion groups, concerts, tours, crafts, exercise options, and more. A movie is offered each evening. If needed, a full-time licensed practical nurse and exercise physiologist are available as well as staff to help with bathing, eating, dressing, and toileting. Donna has been especially enjoying a "well-educated and interesting group of fellow residents" and the frequent special events, such as outings to the theater and local arboretum.

There are approximately 31,000 assisted living facilities in the United States, with four out of five operated for profit. According to my research, over the period from 2004 to 2021, the median annual cost of assisted living has outpaced inflation by 31 percent, increasing to $54,000 per year. Some studies conclude that assisted living facilities have become increasingly focused on maximizing financial gains at the expense of their residents' well-being. That may be true in some cases, but I've heard no complaints from the people I know who reside in such places.

Many people choose board and care homes for old people who are unable to live safely on their own or need help with the chores of daily living. One of my aunts lived in such a place—one that housed just a few people. It was a large house not far from her daughter's home in Colorado. I remember it as being attractive, cheerful, clean, and cozy. She was happy to be there.

Board and care homes typically house 2 to 10 people and offer meals, housekeeping, and help with personal care. Such facilities are licensed by the state and overseen by regulatory agencies. For example, in California, board and care homes are regulated by the California Department of Social Services. To obtain a license for a board and care home, you must receive training, prove financial stability, and meet health and safety requirements, including adequate staffing. Board and care homes differ from assisted living facilities only in their smaller size and in having fewer amenities, such as shared dining rooms, activity rooms and recreational opportunities.

A friend who helped his aunt find a board and care home warned that, in anticipation of your initial visit, the owner or manager might do a bit of staging, such as arranging for the highest-functioning people to be sitting at the breakfast table with newspapers in front of them. Similarly, you might be shown one of the best rooms, only to find later that the room you got was less appealing. When examining board and care homes, he says, "you want the highest functioning level to stimulate your relative." He also recommends talking with the staff to assess their level of engagement with the clients and to learn about staff turnover. In the end, he was satisfied with their choice: "All in all, we had a good experience. The owner-administrator was a person we could easily communicate with and was aware of her special needs."

Nursing homes provide another level of care. They're intended for people needing round-the-clock custodial care, such as bathing, dressing, using the bathroom, eating, and taking medications. *Skilled* nursing facilities offer some medical services, such as rehabilitation, wound care and chronic disease management. The terms for these two types of facilities are often used interchangeably. Hospitals frequently discharge people into nursing homes, a situation I'm familiar with because of visiting friends who needed post-hospital care. I've found these places to be unpleasant, mostly because of the moans and groans emanating from the rooms. Doctor Aronson writes, "Speak human-to-human to most health professionals, and they seem well aware that most nursing homes make a casket look inviting."

Reviews of nursing homes by residents and their families vary widely, as you can see on Yelp. Here are a few comments on one nursing home I'd read about:

> "Trying to find an aide or nurse to answer a question or assist
> with something is a game of hide and seek."

"Totally understaffed. My mom waits and waits."

"The aids are sassy and talk to her like a bad child."

On the brighter side, a reviewer for a place near my home writes that the staff caring for her 96-year-old mother "is attentive and I feel she is in a good home for her next phase of life. [The staff] are dedicated to what they do and it shows. They are professional and compassionate. All the employees get along and have fun together, you can tell the environment is positive and cohesive."

Judging from from my explorations, it looks like you may have to shop around to find a suitable place.

As my firefighter neighbor mentioned, nursing homes frequently call the firehouse to have residents transported to hospitals. The nursing home staff simply don't want to deal with difficult situations, including picking up people who have fallen or ministering to their health needs after a fall. Sarah, a friend who is a nursing student, has worked in nursing homes as part of her training. She tells me, "Typically these facilities are gravely understaffed, leading to lack of individual attention. Frequently the staffing ratios are 24-plus patients to one RN and one or two certified nursing assistants. Call lights go unanswered for long periods of time, by which time the patient is already trying to get up or complete a task without assistance."

Nursing homes are a $100 billion business. The cost of care in nursing homes averages $116,800 annually. A private room in a nursing home costs over $10,000 a month. Medicare generally covers up to 100 days after hospitalization, but long-term care must be paid for out of pocket or through other insurance options. I've learned that about 70 percent of nursing homes are for-profit, and more than half are affiliated with corporate chains. In fact, just five companies own more than 10 percent of the country's 1.7 million licensed nursing-home beds. Private equity has bought up four of the ten largest for-profit nursing homes. Studies have shown that when nursing homes are bought by private-equity groups, frontline nursing staff are cut, and residents are more likely to be hospitalized.

Instead of moving to a facility of one kind or another, many old people move in with their child or other relative. I've found it difficult to separate cases in which the old person is simply cohabiting with the child—often for financial reasons—or is living with their child because, for health reasons, he or she is unable to live alone. I could only find data, from Pew Research, about multigenerational households: "About a quarter of Asian (24%), Black (26%) and Hispanic (26%) Americans lived in multigenerational households in 2021, compared with 13% of those who are White."

Of course, in the past it was much more common for aging parents to live with their children—usually a daughter. That was the case with my grandparents. In her final years, for example, my mother's mother lived with my parents, an arrangement not happily borne by my mother. My father's mother lived with us for a short time when I was sixteen and my sister was away at college. Our two-bedroom, one-bath home was satisfactory for our four-person family, but not for five of us. With my sister at college, my grandma—an immigrant from Russia—shared my bedroom. I hated the arrangement. Grandma used some kind of liniment that permeated the air. Besides, she and I had no fondness for one another. Plus she was grumpy. My sister remembers that she kept lemon drops in her apron pocket but refused to share them with us.

In searching for information about elderly parents living with their adult children, I landed on an AARP web site that included a "comments" section. It was enlightening—maybe even hair-raising. Here are some of the comments written by the old people (grammar and punctuation remain as written):

Unless one is part of the higher income retirees, sharing housing is the most stable housing choice for most of us. Didn't we live together while our children were growing up? I informed my children as they were becoming self-sustaining adults to plan for one of them to have me live with them as I advance in age. All I ask is kitchen privileges and my own room with bath. I won't interfere with their daily activities and could possibly assist financially a bit. I am not their built-in babysitter but I could help in a pinch and I would not impose on them for my needs unless I become incapacitated.

8 years ago, I moved across country to move in with my daughter and SIL [son-in-law]. Best choice we ever made. My quality of life has increased 10 fold, and the grandkids love having grandma around everyday! My daughter and I are closer than ever, and my SIL just told me he is very happy to have me living there in the house. Mind, I won't say we don't have disagreements or things that we get annoyed about. However, we've learned to have mutual respect and to handle issues before they snowball. I would say the key to a successful multi-generational household is communication and respect for each person's privacy and personhood.

I moved in with my oldest daughter and her family when they moved to another state 5 years ago. I am fortunate to say we have had only 3 angry disagreements in that time on topics having nothing to do with our living arrangement. She and my son-in-law do well financially so I don't pay rent or utilities but I contribute in ways to make their lives more manageable so it's a win win. I do not interfere with how they discipline my grand daughter, but she knows GiGi's room is a safe place when sad. I'm an early riser so I get my 7 year old grand daughter ready for school, pack her lunch and drop her off every morning. I make dinner during the week, my daughter cooks on weekends and my son in law does dishes. My daughter and I split the grocery shopping priorities. I shop for everything for my weeknight dinners and my personal needs and she shops for the rest. I babysit when needed and they know they can come and go as they wish if I'm home. After dinner, we part ways and I either visit friends, go play cards or go to my room on the other side of the house where I also have a recliner, 50" TV and computer desk. My older sister doesn't know how we do it........but since my daughter and I have similar outlooks on life, it works! I count my blessings!

I had no choice but take up living with my daughter and her family. I'm trapped because I don't get enough Social Security Disability Benefits to have a place of my own. I'm very unhappy not being able to invite friends from my church to have a bible study, dinner, coffee and cake, or just hang out and watch a movie...they aren't believers. So, I cook, clean house, laundry, babysit 3 boys, and stay in my room. Only outlets are choir practice, Praise Band practice, and church on Sundays. This only alternative has been affecting my health in many ways. When you're a low income, below poverty level senior, choices are very slim. But, it's a choice that's keeping me from being homeless. Looking at all that AARP offers for seniors, I don't see anything that can help me in any way. I may not renew because AARP seems to cater to seniors with money.

As the above quotes imply, adding an elderly parent to your household can be difficult for all parties. The stresses of financial burdens, caretaking, insufficient living space, and incompatibility can lead to serious outcomes. The *Journal of the American Medical Association* reports that "more than 1 of 10 (11%) adults 60 years or older report experiencing at least 1 type of abuse or neglect in the past year." The problem of abuse is exacerbated in cases where the parent has a physical or mental disability. Healthcare professionals are typically mandated to report suspicion of elder maltreatment to Adult Protective Services or other authorities.

But sometimes the abuse can't be laid at the hands of caregivers. The "victim" and the "perpetrator" may be the same person, something *The New England Journal of Medicine* calls "self-neglect"—cases in which the old person exhibits poor judgement, such as not paying bills, misusing alcohol, refusing medical care, refusing a live-in caregiver, and so forth. "Many people of all ages have beliefs or engage in behaviors that lie outside the mainstream, and self-neglect can be difficult to distinguish from a person exercising the right to make choices that many people would consider unwise or unsafe." Such cases pose a dilemma for health care professionals who must try to distinguish self-neglect from abuse.

On a more congenial note, my daughter has friends who can report a more gratifying—though not easy—experience in sharing a home with their elderly mothers. Kim's involvement began with a 2016 Thanksgiving visit to her parents' home in Minnesota. She found that her father, aged 92, was rapidly declining, in part because of liver failure, and her mother had become more forgetful. Kim decided she couldn't leave. She put her career on hold and took over her parents' care, including running the household as well as managing such health matters as monitoring her father's medications and putting in his hearing aids every day. After her father died the following July, she decided to stay with her mother until she and her two brothers could arrange to move her mother to Washington State where they lived. Four and a half years later, Kim was still living with her mother in Minnesota. In 2018, her mother fell and broke her arms. The following year she developed a pulmonary embolism and fell again. Then Covid hit. "The winter of 20/21," Kim says, "found me a bit desperate." It was time to move.

With the help of her brothers and their wives, her mother's house was sold, and both Kim and her mother moved to Kim's brother's farm in northern Washington. "Mom was not pleased to move but was stoically compliant." For Kim, the arrangement was a "big relief after being alone with her for four-and-a-half years in Minnesota." At the farm, Kim was her mother's main caregiver, which included managing her medications, making doctor appointments, and accompanying her mother to them. But, Kim says, her mother's care was a "group effort." For example, her sister-in-law did the cooking. To provide some weekday hours "free of monitoring/being available to her," the family hired an aide to come for half a day, Monday through Friday, at a cost of $3,000 a month, which was paid for by her father's long-term health insurance.

After more than three years, Kim's mother was resettled to an Adult Family Home near a brother who lives in suburban Seattle, an arrangement that has been satisfactory for both her mother and Kim. (Adult Family

Homes are community-based residences that are licensed and regulated by the state of Washington to provide 24-hour care and daily living services. Each home is independently licensed and operated and can serve between two and six residents. Costs for a private room start at $5,000 a month.) As Kim says, "I have recovered a lot of my agency, no longer being her primary caregiver. I see her two times a week now (she's 45 minutes from me) and I feel lighter and more focused and engaged with her and can deal with the short-term (shorter and shorter) memory loss much better, not living and caretaking 24/7. I cherish her more and more. We go to the library and get ice cream regularly. She sees her great-grandkids and my brother and sister-in-law regularly. She's made peace with her new scene and is grateful. She puzzles, does social media, magazines (can't stay with a book plot) and watches TV." At the time of this writing, Kim's mother was 94.

A second example of a congenial arrangement comes from Lanna, another friend of my daughter's. After Lanna's father died, her mother, Margaret, continued to live in Arizona—the first time living by herself. But her home was over 500 miles away from any of her children, and, after three years, Margaret was getting lonely and ready to live with one of her children, where she was clearly welcome. As Lanna described it, her sister Joni "immediately called dibs on her, but it was agreed that she would spend the winter months in Florida and the summer months in Nevada with me. This was to give her the best climate year-round and to give my sister and me time to be on our own." This two-state arrangement worked well for all parties, but after ten years, Margaret found it increasingly difficult to prepare for and make the trips back and forth. At age 95, she decided that her next flight was to be her last. Because Joni's health had been deteriorating, the sisters agreed that their mother would reside with Lanna.

As she had in her previous visits, Margaret will continue to reside in the guest room, which she had furnished and decorated herself. Because winters are cold where Lanna lives, and because her mother gets cold easily, Lanna says she'll be "keeping the house warmer than we're used to and spending more on heating bills." Margaret pays them $1,000 a month to cover rent, food and utilities, an amount she set herself and that "has worked out fine for everybody so far."

Lanna notes that her mother is healthy for her age. "Her major health issues are hearing loss and deteriorating eyesight (macular degeneration) which is getting noticeably worse." Lanna accompanies her mother to medical appointments, which has become increasingly important. As Lanna says, her mother "has tended to not understand or fully remember what was discussed. I think she often doesn't hear everything and then doesn't ask questions or have anything repeated."

According to Lanna, her mother "spends all of her time in her room in her comfortable chair...but is never really doing nothing." She reads, plays electronic games on her iPad, watches TV, and plays board games and dominoes with Lanna. She checks her bank account every day and her credit card frequently and still "does a great job managing her finances."

Margaret rarely goes out except for a once-a-week trip to get her hair done. As Lanna says, "She is very conscious of her appearance and comes out every morning with hair and makeup done and dressed in a nice outfit." Overall, though, Margaret "is pretty much socially isolated except for some visits from extended family members and infrequent telephone calls with some old friends. She seems to like it that way." Margaret no longer joins Lanna and her husband for restaurant dinners. Such outings require too much effort, and noisy restaurants make hearing impossible.

Even though her mother has been generally self-sufficient, Lanna has noticed that it's become increasingly difficult for her to walk even a short distance.

> "So even though no specific plans have been made, we will be looking into some possible in-home care and other services related to her vision in the near future and will also be ready for moving her to assisted living if and when I'm unable to meet all her physical needs. She is quite resistant to having anyone come stay with her or help her in any way really. I've brought it up with her, of course, and get resistance or silence. I am going to find someone who she can become comfortable with and will have be firm about it so that I can have a few opportunities to get away and also have the help for myself."

As to Lanna's own well-being, she writes—

> I have struggled at times with not having the freedom to plan trips or just weekends away and I am more worried about that now that she'll be here full time. My Mom and I get along very well but are opposites when it comes to politics or religion so those things are avoided. But life happens and those important value-based topics do creep in when you're together so much. She can be stubborn, narrow-minded and judgmental (traits I have longstanding issues about). At this point in my life, I am comfortable with who I am and what I believe so I stay true to myself while keeping things on an even keel. I never thought I would be in a position where

we would live together full time because she and Joni have much more in common so I would have guessed she would be with Joni. It's been clear for a long time that it wasn't going that way and I've adjusted to the idea over time. I love my Mom and do enjoy her company. She could afford to live in an assisted living facility instead of here and I know she would do that in a heartbeat if her being here was a problem for me. I would rather have her with me as long as I can provide what she needs and she feels the same. I know for now that this is the best place for her.

At the time of this writing, Lanna and my daughter had arranged to attend a workshop together after which they were both going to come visit my husband and me for a couple of nights. The plan was for Margaret to stay at home in the capable hands of Lanna's husband. But, while still at the workshop, Lanna got word that Margaret had become anxious about Lanna's absence. Lanna went straight home from the workshop.

Dr. Aronson concludes, "When asked the recipe for a good old age, I often give a list: good genes, good luck, enough money, and one good kid, usually a daughter."

For old people without a family member to take them in or the means to pay for housing, living on the streets is increasingly becoming their only option. As one of the commenters on the AARP website wrote, "When you're a low income, below poverty level senior, choices are very slim. But, it's a choice [living with a child] that's keeping me from being homeless." In fact, many people who are 65 and over are homeless. Their number has reached a record high of 70,000. In an odd parent-living-with child reversal, one out of eight people aged 65 and over became homeless when their parents died. This cohort entered the workforce amid recessions and a shift to a post-industrial economy. Because of low-wage jobs and high housing costs, many depended on their parents for financial help and a place to live. As social scientist Dennis Culhane at the University of Pennsylvania notes, "You have a generation of adult children who depend on their parents because they can't afford housing on their own. When their parents die, they have no place to live. We're seeing more and more of them on the streets and in shelters."

It may seem that the wide variety of living arrangements for old people provide plenty of options. But if you haven't the means or family support, your choices are reduced to nearly zero. Count yourself lucky if you have the luxury of choosing.

Chapter Ten

Caregiving

Most old people—64 percent—get care from their children, spouses, other relatives, or non-relatives. According to the U.S. Bureau of Labor Statistics, approximately 38.2 million people provide unpaid care to the elderly. That's 14 percent of the U.S. population age 15 and above (2023-2024). Most caregivers need to balance their jobs with caregiving duties. Many have had to quit work or shift from full-time to part-time work. A quarter of America's 40 million unpaid caregivers are themselves over age 75, and most are women.

"Caring for seniors, while a labor of love, can nonetheless be grinding," writes Michelle Cottle in *The New York Times*. "It is often compared to parenting, but the emotional and cultural space it occupies is very different. With a frail parent, there is no sense of guiding someone toward a bright future. Quite the opposite." She describes her caregiving experience as a "journey—and not a low-key pleasure trip with a clear itinerary you can plan and pack for." Rather, she writes, "...my family's caregiving experience spiraled into a chaotic spectacle that was part harrowing medical drama, part sitcom. Even early on, there were 2 a.m. phone calls, mangled medical equipment, emergency room visits, dizzying medication schedules...."

As Dr. Aronson notes, "Caregiving is hard work. More often than not, it's tedious, awkwardly intimate, physically exhausting and emotionally challenging. Sometimes it is also dangerous or disgusting. Almost always it is 24/7...and has profound adverse health consequences for those who do it. It is women's work and immigrants' work, and it is work that we have made so undesirable and difficult that many people either can't or won't do it."

More than sixteen million Americans provide uncompensated care for people with dementias, a particularly difficult task. My sister-in-law, Mary, was the caregiver for her husband, Bill. His dementia became noticeable in 2010 when, she writes, "he began to ask me the same questions over again in a short span of time or would forget to run an errand I had requested." His first diagnosis was "mild cognitive impairment." His disease progressed and his symptoms worsened with each year. To make life easier, Mary and Bill moved to an assisted living facility that gave Bill "access to social activities and allowed him a certain amount of freedom." After a few years, they relocated to a continuing care retirement community (CCRC) that offered a memory care facility on the same grounds, although Mary chose to keep him at home, taking care of all of his needs, including such ministrations as helping him shower and dress, and trimming his nails.

In the last months of Bill's life, Mary had help from hospice and home care aides who came in for a few hours a day. Hospice supplied a hospital bed, special supplies and medications as well as a nurse who checked in once a week. A hospice doctor was available when needed. (I was surprised to learn that, to qualify for hospice, Mary had to terminate their relationship with their primary care doctor.) Most helpful to Mary were the aides she hired through a private company. Not only did they come for a few hours every day to perform routine tasks, such as bathing and bed changing, but they also gave Mary "some peace of mind and a little freedom." Medicare covered hospice care. Bill's long-term health insurance covered the cost of the other aides.

In 2022, 12 years after his initial diagnosis, Bill died of its complications following a fall. Near the end, as his condition worsened, Mary recalls calling hospice one evening, telling them she was concerned that "Bill's breathing rate was very rapid. What does this mean? How can I help him?" She was told the rapid breathing means that he's dying and he would probably die in the next few hours. She was also told that when he died to call back and they would send a doctor to come and pronounce him dead. "It was all quite matter of fact." Mary was stunned. Nevertheless, as predicted, Bill died later that night.

"One of the biggest frustrations with this disease," Mary says,

> is that no one can tell you, the caregiver, what to expect. Every patient is different. There is no certain prognosis like in most diseases. There is not a lot of emotional support for caregivers, especially not from the medical profession. One of the best support persons I had the last year of Bill's life was my next-door neighbor. She also had a husband with dementia. Most mornings we would sit on my front porch and compare notes, information, and just generally be a support to one another. Our husbands died four days apart in 2022. This disease has been called 'the long goodbye.' I had lost Bill, but I had been losing him slowly for 12 years. I knew I had taken good care of him. I could take solace in that.

In sharing her story, Mary told me that her friend and neighbor, who was also her husband's caretaker, found it disheartening to deal with what she calls "flyover visitors": people, including her husband's adult children, who would come for a visit and stay just long enough to get a favorable impression of her situation. For these visits, her husband, who had Alzheimer's disease, would manage to "hold it together" just long enough to leave the impression with the visitors that all was well, giving them no inkling of her long-haul, day-to-day struggles.

In a similar vein, a blogger I'd heard about shared his experiences of caring for his wife who also has Alzheimer's disease. Like Mary, he notes that "there are no rules or a set guide for the family caregiver to follow." He also laments lack of support: "Most of my 'best lifelong friends' and some of my wife's family members have vanished during the Alzheimer's. They have no idea of my lifestyle as a 24/7 home caregiver and my wife's behavioral changes with this disease." He also writes how his fear, anger, and sadness vie for control over his "soul and spirit," finding it incredibly difficult to balance these "dreadful feelings with others, such as hope, love, and happiness."

Another caregiver, my sister's friend, Cheryl, is in her 70s and was the caregiver for her husband. She writes—

"Does my wife know I'm here?" my husband of 40 years asked me as we were climbing into bed. I laughed. He didn't. That was the moment I knew his MCI (Mild Cognitive Impairment) was morphing into the uncharted waters of full-blown dementia. During the ensuing seven years we were tossed about in the murkiness of a health care system that was devoid of both *care* and a functional *system*. Eventually, we landed in the office of a competent neurologist who did a meticulous review of my husband's medical records, performed a two-hour exam and diagnosed him as having Alzheimer's. All in one day. A map to navigate the future course.

Now as a "seasoned" caregiver, I can tell you that if you ever inherit this type of responsibility, you will know inevitable heartbreaks, stupefying exhaustion, confusion, frustration and self-doubt. And, if lucky, you might experience the grace of unexpected resilience, ingenuity, intelligence and energy that surfaces inexplicably when needed most. Below are pearls I have gleaned along the way:

Devoted and trusted friends are your life jackets.
Humor is your raft.
Never hesitate to signal SOS.
Trust your intuition.
Every day presents a new learning curve.
Guilt is a self-indulgent undertow.

There is a dizzying wealth of resources available that seem to emerge daily: online support groups, podcasts, books, blogs, newsletters, organizations etc. I perused them obsessively but in retrospect I might have been better served by spending more time in my hammock with a cozy mystery.

For user-friendly and practical advice, Cheryl recommends Teepa Snow, an occupational therapist and dementia care educator that you can find on YouTube, as well as the following books:
Surviving Alzheimer's by Paula Spencer Scott
The Caregiver's Guide to Dementia by Gail Weatherill
The 36-Hour Day by Nancy L. Mace and Peter V. Rabins

Loving Someone Who Has Dementia by Pauline Boss

I have a friend, Betsy, whose daughter Alice served as her caregiver twice, once in 2018 following a horrific car accident when Betsy was 73, and once in 2024 after a fall. I was impressed to learn that Alice had prepared herself to be a caregiver long before she was needed. In fact, it started when she took a Death and Dying class in college, where she learned the importance of designating a primary caregiver as one way of avoiding family breakups that can occur in the process of making life-and-death decisions for a family member. Alice says, "I wanted to ensure that didn't occur within our family, so I asked my mother decades ago if I could be designated as primary caregiver."

Alice's preparedness turned out to be a godsend when, years later, Betsy was hit head-on by a drug-addled, uninsured driver. Her injuries were extensive and included a severely broken ankle that required a six-hour surgery, as well as five broken ribs, bruised lung tissue, a broken tailbone, and a broken sternum. Alice arrived at the ER with a printout of her mother's insurance information, which she keeps in her wallet. After that, her caregiving duties began in earnest, as she explains:

> During the aftermath of the car accident, I interfaced with the insurance company regarding what would be required for them related to coverage for her injuries and totaled car. I was in touch with her health insurance companies regarding coverage for her tens of thousands of ER, ICU, and rehabilitation facility bills. I also obtained a personal injury attorney, as we needed guidance and expertise regarding how to handle the insurance companies and how to make sure they didn't find ways to shirk delivering on her benefits and coverage.

Within a day of her accident, I also emailed as many of her friends and family members that I could find emails for, letting them know what had happened. I continued to interface with many people who wanted to support her and visit her over the next many weeks.

The rehab facility personnel were wonderful in many ways, but the food was abysmal. So, I regularly bought and delivered meals and snacks that could be kept in the refrigerator for her. A few times I brought her a warm meal from a restaurant.

I also met with the occupational nurse at my mother's house in preparation for her return home, to make sure it was appropriately safe for her as she returned in a wheelchair, with recovery and pain still ahead of her.

Six years later, when Betsy took a fall and injured her back, Alice was surprised to learn that, even though her mother's injuries were far less serious than those she suffered in the car accident, "caregiving was actually more challenging, as I drove her into the ER three times in one week, hoping she would not fall as she hobbled with a walker across the wet driveway to the car." Alice also found herself performing the duties that had been previously carried out by rehabilitation professionals in the facility where Betsy had resided for ten weeks following the car accident. That is, she had to help Betsy shower, ensure that she could safely get to the bathroom, and make certain that she had a stock of easy-to-prepare meals.

"The day-to-day caregiving this time was much more intense," Alice says.

> Trying to navigate and coordinate her surgery, her meals, her many doctor appointments, her pain medication, and, ultimately, creating and managing a calendar full of daily in-home appointments with nurses, PTs, OTs, took a LOT of time and energy to manage. (Although I would be remiss without mentioning the extreme help that the Visiting Nurses Association provided as she recovered. Having in-home medical appointments was vital, as any time I had to take her in-person to an appointment posed a risk of another fall, as she was experiencing dizziness and instability.)

Pain management was especially challenging for Alice. After the 2018 event, nurses in the ICU and rehab managed Betsy's pain levels and medications. In 2024, Alice and Betsy were in charge of controlling Betsy's pain and ensuring that the medications were properly dosed and available when needed. Because prescriptions for controlled substances limit the number of pills allotted, and it can take up to 72 hours to obtain a prescription renewal, Alice found that helping Betsy manage her pain was an especially stressful endeavor. To reduce the stress, Alice created a table of Betsy's medications, complete with checkboxes for Betsy to record her doses. She created a similar table for Betsy to keep track of her physical therapy exercises and repetitions. "All of this," Alice admits, "was, frankly, stressful and consuming."

Alice and Betsy occasionally found themselves engaged in what Alice describes as power struggles, with Alice trying to ensure Betsy's safety from harm, and Betsy trying to be less of a burden by taking on more housekeeping chores, such as the laundry. Similar disagreements centered on Alice's keeping tabs on Betsy's adherence to her physical therapy routines.

Were it not for the fact that Alice lives directly behind her mother and works a flexible job, her comprehensive caregiving—along with the attendant tug of wars—would not have been possible.

Endless caregiving, especially in isolation, has a negative impact on the caregiver's health. It can raise blood pressure, disrupt sleep, and trigger anxiety and depression. One fifth of those caring for the elderly report that their health has deteriorated because of it. The deterioration includes an increase in inflammation, which contributes to age-related bodily damage. In a study released by the CDC in 2024, caregivers scored worse than noncaregivers on 13 of 19 health indicators. Because of increased inflammation, caregivers appear biologically older than those without the caregiving burden. The root cause is chronic stress, which hampers the immune system. One study, conducted at Ohio State University, found that spouses caring for ill partners recovered more slowly from puncture wounds on their arms than those who weren't providing care.

Thirty-seven percent of caregivers report burnout. They're forced to confront their limits, and, because they're immersed in a daily routine of essential human needs, it can also make them feel out of step with other people—that their old sense of self as a worker, spouse, parent or friend doesn't match up to what they do all day. They find this disconnect makes them feel disoriented, lost, or alone. As one caregiver said, "I think it's a transformation for everybody, and it's permanent. This idea that you'll go back to the person you were before, that's never going to happen."

As to paid caregivers, home care is among the fastest-growing occupations. In 2024, the number of home health aides and personal care aides rose to 3.2 million, up from 1.4 million a decade earlier. At this writing, there was a shortage of workers, a problem that's driven partly by low wages. The median hourly wage for all care workers was $16.72 in 2023—lower than the wage for all other jobs with similar or low entry-level requirements. That wage, however, is not what consumers pay the home care agencies, which typically charge $34.00 an hour. Michelle Cottle reported that the cost of the aides she hired to care for her father came to about $3,500 per week, paid "out of pocket from the get-go, since neither Medicare nor private health insurance typically covers most long-term care costs."

Current estimates suggest that the direct care worker shortage will grow to 860,000 by 2032, and that 8.9 million positions will need to be filled over the next decade to meet the demand. Immigrants make up 28 percent of the long-term-care workforce, a figure that's been rising in recent years. Caregiving professionals have noted that foreign-born workers tend to re-gard looking after seniors as desirable, meaningful work. Many come from cultures that revere their elders. *The New England Journal of Medicine* notes that "immigrants are a vital part of the U.S. Health care system: at least one in five U.S. health care workers is foreign-born, including 29% of physicians, 17% of nurses, and 24% of direct care workers;...of the 37% of foreign-born direct care workers who are noncitizens, nearly half may be undocumented."

Raids by ICE have made matters worse. As the *Journal* noted, "Just four days after the inauguration, 25 undocumented Filipino direct care workers were arrested in an ICE raid at a senior care facility in Chicago; at least eight have been deported." In one case, a cancer patient, living alone at home, had fallen but wasn't found for days because "his home health aide had stopped coming to work for fear of deportation." Non-immigrants are unlikely to fill the void. Direct care workers "are often subject to ex-ploitative work practices, including wage theft. The physically demanding nature of direct care work, combined with low pay and high susceptibility to exploitation, makes these roles unattractive to U.S.-born and highly skilled foreign-born workers."

Even with the low wages, many families cannot afford to pay for caregivers. As Dr. Aronson notes, "In twenty years of geriatrics, I had only met a handful of working- or lower-middle-class families who had been able to find an American willing to care for their aging relative for a salary they could afford."

I'm lucky that I've never been required to be a caregiver or needed one for myself—yet. As I mentioned in the Introduction, both of my parents died instantly from heart attacks—not at the same time—while they were still living independently. My husband doesn't need a caregiver. If I am ever required to be a caregiver, I'll look to Mary and Cheryl as role models. Both were in their 70s when caring for their husbands, and both took on the task with grace, compassion, intelligence, and dedication.

Chapter Eleven

Health care

We old people frequently need health care. After all, we're breaking down. In fact, we account for 37 percent of health care spending.

I seek medical help when I have a problem I can't fix myself, most recently a laceration in my leg that needed stitches. (When opening the car door, I managed to smash it into my lower leg.) I went to an urgent care center—about a 40-minute drive from my home. It wasn't convenient, but my husband was home so he could drive me while I managed my bleeding leg. I'm lucky that I don't have any chronic conditions requiring regular visits to healthcare providers. But my occasional emergencies provide enough exposure to allow me to speak from experience.

Speaking for myself and others in my aging cohort, I think it's safe to say that we have had both positive and negative experiences with doctors and medical institutions—their competency, availability, and costs. The negative experiences are caused partly by doctors' attitudes toward old people, and partly by our dysfunctional healthcare system.

Let's start with the doctors themselves. In his book, *Being Mortal*, Dr. Atul Gawande tells us that a lot of doctors don't like taking care of the elderly: "They hardly know what to do and often only make matters worse.

…Taking care of a debilitated, elderly person in our medicalized era is an overwhelming combination of the technological and the custodial."

In *Elderhood*, geriatrician Louise Aronson tells us that geriatrics is of little interest to medical students. Not only is the number of doctors who choose geriatric medicine small, but their salaries tend to be $20,000 less than other specialties. Agism is also a factor, as evidenced by a remark made by a medical student's mentor that Aronson overheard: "Unless you really like changing adult diapers, don't waste your time learning geriatrics." No wonder there's a shortage of geriatricians!

Adam Kay, who was once a doctor in the British National Health Service and is now a writer, says, in his book, *Undoctored,* "There is a clear invisibility to the very elderly, where we fail to see them as people with at least twice our lived existence….Medicine is often guilty of letting the elderly blend into an amorphous homogeneity—wrinkled bags of skin and warfarin [a blood thinner]."

Doctors find us uninteresting unless we have a discrete problem they can fix. Dr. Gawande himself admits that he has "encountered patients forced to confront the realities of decline and mortality, and it did not take long to realize how unready I was to help them." Doctor Aronson adds that among the reasons doctors cite for not liking to take care of old patients "is the moral distress they feel when they are asked to provide futile treatments that cause significant suffering."

It seems that we old people are both uninteresting and threatening to doctors' sense of their own ability to help. Moreover, as one medical student comments, "doctors assume that when an old person comes in there's going to be a ton of problems and it's going to be a pain to address all those issues." I can't say I blame medical students for not choosing geriatrics. I don't think I would either.

Whether you're old or not, research has shown that most physicians already have in mind two or three diagnoses within minutes of meeting a patient. Many don't listen to the patients' complaints. I think that's particularly true if you're old. A 1999 study of 29 family physician practices found that doctors let patients speak for only 23 seconds before redirecting them. Only one in four patients got to finish his or her statement before being interrupted. A segment of the PBS News Hour provided this example: A woman with an acute sinus infection went to see an ear-nose-and throat specialist who, she said, "...looked up my nose, said it was inflamed, told me to see the nurse for a prescription and was gone." When she began to question the doctor's choice of medication, "He just cut me off totally," she said. "I've never been in and out from a visit faster." My sister, at age 88, went to a pulmonologist who never talked with her, touched her, or examined her lung capacity. Instead, he sent her to a clerk to arrange a lung biopsy, which she refused. Even if a doctor listens to your account of a problem, they often ignore your words, mostly, I suppose, because they are the experts and you are not.

More than the doctors themselves, it's the structure of our health care system that shortchanges us. Seventy percent of doctors work as salaried employees of large hospital systems or corporate entities, taking orders from administrators and executives who do not always share their values or priorities. For example, because of the insurance reimbursement requirements and/or strictures imposed by their medical institutions, doctors must rush through examinations, as was the case for the sinus sufferer above. They may also be pressured to make decisions based on financial considerations. The emphasis is on speed, efficiency, and relative value units (R.V.U.s.), a metric that rewards doctors for doing tests and procedures and discourages them from spending too much time on less remunerative functions, such as listening and talking to patients. In the eyes of their patients, doctors may become scapegoats—the instruments of betrayal by the health care system.

It's no surprise that doctors are increasingly suffering from burnout. In the opinion of Dr. Eric Reinhart, a physician at Northwestern University, burnout is caused in large part by "...our dwindling faith in the systems for which we work." Definitions of burnout have included emotional exhaustion in response to intensive work, becoming emotionally drained, detachment from and negative feelings toward people they are trying to help, and a sense of helplessness and loss of purpose.

Nearly two-thirds of physicians report that they are "...finding it difficult to quash the suspicion that our institutions, and much of our work inside them, primarily serve a moneymaking machine." Examples include hospitals putting profits over people, the use of billing codes that dictate nearly every aspect of medical practice, and the profit motives of insurance and pharmaceutical companies—all barriers to improving patients' lives. A study of 10,000 family physicians showed that key contributors to burnout include the lack of a fully-staffed support team and the amount of time they must spend at home working on electronic health records.

This situation has been taking a toll for years. The suicide rate among doctors is higher than the rate among active military members. One in five health care workers has quit his or her job since the start of the pandemic, and an additional 31 percent have considered leaving. In the remarks of some doctors: "Every day, you're reminded how savage the system is"; "It's turned us into a widget factory of just throughput, getting people in, getting people transferred onto money-making specialties, without really addressing their health care needs. And it's demoralizing and it's not good care."

Palliative care doctors—those who care for patients at the end of their lives—often find themselves in precarious positions, walking a line between their own security and vulnerability. Sometimes they're fired by patients and their families who are unhappy with their treatment. As one palliative care doctor reported in the *Journal of the American Medical Association*, the cause for dismissals is because

> We invite difficult conversations, confront people with news they prefer to avoid, and encourage otherwise taboo topics such as human frailty and death. Our focus on what may go wrong differs from other clinicians' optimism and may be unwelcome to patients and health care teams alike. We acknowledge emotional vulnerability, explore uncertainty, uncover fears, and describe a future in which patients make difficult choices about how they live and how they die.

Here are some examples of why he and other palliative care doctors were fired: asking if a suicidal patient had access to a gun; asking "intrusive questions"; supporting a family's decision to discontinue life-sustaining therapies for a loved one with multiple organ failure; sharing the impression that a patient with cancer was dying (the family preferred the oncologist's version of a more hopeful future).

Palliative care doctors are in a difficult position. The way they're perceived and rated by patients varies according to how they communicate an unfavorable prognosis. In a randomized trial of 100 patients with advanced cancer, study participants viewed videos of encounters between patients and oncologists who expressed either optimistic or realistic outcomes. The study revealed that participants perceived the optimistic oncologists as more compassionate and trustworthy, even if the information they shared was misleading. Another study of nearly 1,200 patients with advanced cancer found that satisfaction with a doctor's communication skills was inversely associated with the accuracy of the doctor's prognosis. In other words, the study found that the harder a doctor tried to make the patient understand the seriousness of his or her condition, the less satisfied the patient was with the doctor's care. Taken together, these and other studies suggest that patients like and trust those clinicians who provide optimistic outlooks more than those whose outlooks are more realistic.

Now we have a chronic physician shortage. One in five doctors plans to stop practicing in the coming years. In 2021, about 117,000 physicians left the work force, while fewer than 40,000 joined it. According to projections published by the Association of American Medical Colleges, the United States will face a physician shortage of up to 86,000 physicians by 2036. Twenty-nine percent of physicians in the U.S. were not born here, demonstrating our need for immigrant healthcare workers.

Even though there's a shortage of primary care doctors, multibillion-dollar corporations are gobbling up primary care practices. For example, CVS paid $11 billion to buy a chain of primary care centers. Primary care practices are valuable because the doctors oversee vast numbers of patients and thus have the potential to bring business and profits to hospital systems, health insurers, and/or pharmacies. Now, nearly 7 in 10 of all doctors, including my GP, are employed by either a hospital or a corporation. This type of consolidation is driven by the quest for profits, not patients' welfare.

My own experience is an example of what happens when corporations take over primary care practices. For 50 years, our small town (population 5,000) had a medical clinic—a private practice that had been established by a beloved local doctor. It was a five-minute drive from our house to the clinic. We could drop in and be seen. Then, in 2006, Dignity Health Medical Group bought the practice. In 2023, they shut it down and moved the doctors to offices a half-hour's drive away.

A year or so after our local clinic closed, I discovered a tick buried in the flabby part of my upper underarm. My husband tried removing the tick with our special tools but was unable to extract the tick's entire body. Its head was still lodged in my arm. Because I tend to believe my body will heal itself, I considered leaving it there, but the next day I changed my mind. My upper arm had become red, swollen, and sore. Because we no longer have a nearby clinic, I thought I might go to a new—rather dysfunctional—clinic that had opened in the town next to ours. Their website said the office was open, so I drove there, only to find that they were not, in fact, open.

Next, I drove to the Dignity Health office where my GP is now based. It was my first visit to that office, which is located in a strip mall with limited parking. The office is tastefully decorated in Dignity's signature color scheme. Two receptionists sat behind tall counters tapping at their computers. I asked if someone could remove the tick's head from my arm. Answer: "We don't take walk-ins." With that, they directed me to a Dignity-owned urgent care office, located in a beach town another half-hour's drive away. I was able to find it using my GPS. When I got there, the nurse wanted to take my blood pressure. I refused, but he insisted, so I gave in. Big mistake. It was over 200, no surprise, considering my ordeal. After the doctor removed the tick part—it took about two minutes—he encouraged me to stay in the office until they could bring my blood pressure down. His exact words were: "You could die on the way home." I told him I felt fine and left. That evening, I took my blood pressure. It was normal for me: 137 systolic (upper number). (I don't remember the lower, diastolic, number).

Here's another Dignity story written by my sister, Elaine. When she was 88, she'd been having unexplained bouts of fatigue. To diagnose this situation, her GP recommended some tests at the Cardiovascular Diagnostic Center of Dignity Health in Prescott, Arizona, where Elaine lives. After a two-week wait she arrived for her appointment. As she tells it,

Don and I entered through a large automatic door to find an enormous glass room buzzing with staff. Nearby were a myriad of chairs filled with waiting clients looking as confused as I was. I approached the wide desk, manned by several harried people, and told them why I was there. They sent me to the second floor. This required a ride on an elevator whose buttons were so obscure we couldn't find them.

Eventually we found our floor and were directed down a long hallway (while I'm thinking of heart patients more feeble than I). We came to another huge, glassed area with a bleak, sterile atmosphere. Again, we had to trek down a long hall past another crowd of people in chairs before arriving at a reception cubicle behind glass.

Then began the sign-in. I was required to sign in while I stood at a computer that I couldn't make work properly. Don assisted and finally—with the help of a man in one of the chairs—we managed. Behind her glass and desk, the impatient receptionist gave me an ID bracelet and ordered me to wait. We sat for a while, and I was then ushered down another hall by a tech.

The tech looked me over, including at my walking stick, and she and her partner agreed that they wanted an OK before administering the stress test on a treadmill. They consulted a doc down the hall who didn't emerge from an office, and that invisible person decided the stress test wasn't safe for me.

They sent me home.

Later, Elaine's GP received an email from the Dignity people. The message said, "Patient refuses to get on the treadmill."

As these examples show, corporate medicine can make visits to health care providers difficult for old people to navigate. Of course, it's not only old people who find our healthcare system frustrating. The obstacles—such as discovering that the surgeon who sewed you up was "out of network" (not covered by your insurance) or that your treatment required "prior authorization" from insurers—affect people of all ages.

To make matters worse, not only are corporations buying primary care practices, but private equity firms are purchasing hospitals in increasing numbers. Since 2008, American hospitals have been involved in more than a thousand mergers and acquisitions, resulting in large, powerful health systems that influence both the price of hospital care and the reimbursement rates paid by private insurers. In recent years, 66 billion dollars was spent on acquisitions, a situation that has led to price hikes and unnecessary procedures.

At the time of this writing, private equity firms owned 30 percent of all hospitals, a situation that results in negative health outcomes for patients. As reported in the *Journal of the American Medical Association*, researchers compared private equity and non-private equity hospitals. They found that, after the hospitals were purchased by private equity firms, the rates of hospital-acquired complications for patients increased by 25 percent. The increase was driven by a 27 percent increase in falls; a 38 percent increase in central line infections, which are associated with ICU care; and a doubling of surgical site infections. Clearly, money-saving measures are detrimental to patient health and safety.

Even though I'm critical of our healthcare system, I'm grateful to occasionally get help, especially when I find a talented and competent doctor to fix what ails me. This happened when I was 88 and had been experiencing severe sciatic pain that ran from my hip to my foot. I'd tried physical therapy, chiropractic, and even acupuncture. Nothing helped. Perhaps surgery was required. Then I remembered meeting a neurosurgeon—a woman—after she'd performed a muscle biopsy on my husband (he had been suffering from severe muscle weakness and pain in his arms and legs, a side effect of a drug he'd been taking for colitis). After the biopsy, when she came out to greet me, I told her about the drug prescribed for his colitis and its consequences. She said, "That's why I don't take pills."

Because of that brief encounter, I remembered her years later when I decided to seek a surgeon for my sciatic pain. I called her office, hoping to make an appointment. Of course, that was not possible. First, I had to get a referral from my GP, an annoying requirement that requires an extra doctor visit (and strikes me as extortion). After finally meeting with the neurosurgeon and getting an MRI and X-rays, she recommended a laminectomy—a procedure to remove a bit of bone, the lamina, that was pressing on my sciatic nerve. The surgery required a two-inch incision and some drilling. I went home a few hours after the procedure. Relief was instant and, so far, permanent. Moreover, I was able to return to my normal routines after only a week or so.

Like me, many of us have had successful outcomes from medical treatments and are grateful for them. At the same time, experts agree that our healthcare system needs fixing, especially considering the growing population of old people. A recent *Nature Portfolio* journal tells us our healthcare system is on the brink: "The United States is undergoing a demographic and health transformation that will have profound implications for its healthcare system and society....With an aging population requiring more care and a strained system facing workforce shortages, capacity issues, and fragmentation, innovative solutions and policy reforms are needed." As to demographic transformations, another recent journal article states that "by 2050, women 75 and older will be the largest age subgroup in the US."

Experts everywhere agree that we need more medical personnel trained in geriatrics—people who are fluent in the basics: evaluating functional status, managing falls and delirium, and conducting advanced care planning. According to a 2025 article in the journal *JAMA Network Open*, there is, in fact, a growing movement to prepare all physicians to care for old people. National initiatives, the journal reports, are encouraging hospitals and clinics to "meet specific benchmarks for elder care," and to "hardwire what good care should look like" for older patients.

At the same time, we're far short of the estimated 20,000 geriatricians needed to meet the nation's current needs. Even though research has shown substantial declines in the percentage of medical schools requiring geriatrics clerkships (hands-on training in a specialty), the schools nevertheless recognize the importance of training medical students in the unique health care needs of old people. As reported in the journal *Academic Medicine*, a working group of the American Geriatrics Society has developed a set of competencies in geriatric medicine. They call these competencies the 5Ms, encouraging practitioners to focus on—

- Multicomplexity—the whole person living with multiple chronic conditions, advanced illness, and/or with complicated needs that may include the interaction of biological, psychological, and social factors.

- Mind—thinking, remembering, reasoning, dementia, delirium, depression.

- Mobility—amount of mobility, function, impaired gait and balance, fall injury prevention.

- Medications—polypharmacy and deprescribing, optimal prescribing, adverse medications effects, medication burden.

- What Matters Most—each individual's own meaningful health outcome goals and care preferences.

These initiatives are a step in the right direction. Whether they become widespread practices remains to be seen.

Chapter Twelve

Advocacy

When we're in need of medical treatment, we may find ourselves face to face with a provider explaining the fine points of our ailments, such as, in my case, lumbar radiculopathy, lumbar stenosis, and degenerative scoliosis (pinched nerve, narrowing of the spinal canal, and curved spine, respectively). The provider may also discuss treatment options, next steps, and what to expect. It's a lot to take in, especially if we have dementia or hearing loss. We need to make decisions, and we want to be sure our decisions are right for us.

Doctor Aronson says,

> Absent any direction, the default position of the American health care system is to "do everything." More often than not, this approach does not actually include "everything," since it so rarely includes essential conversations about a person's future, care designed to minimize distress and maximize comfort, information about likely life expectancy, and options for treatment in a familiar environment. Each of those approaches...is generally not provided in today's technology-obsessed and profit-driven health systems.

Hence, the need for advocates. An advocate is someone who assists patients in navigating the healthcare system, including ensuring the patient understands medical conditions and treatment options, monitoring care, and finding qualified healthcare providers.

Connie Burgess, RN, has wide-ranging experience with health care, having served in nearly every hospital department, from ob-gyn to hospice as well as the ICU. Because she has often witnessed the barriers we face when engaging with health care providers, I asked her to give me her insider's views and recommendations regarding advocacy.

For one thing, she says, advocates are needed because many providers lack expertise in geriatrics. She has also seen agism or cultural biases that "lead to undervalued needs and preferences of elderly patients." Moreover, she tells me, physicians may regard us as too old to benefit from further treatment, or they may hold misogynistic beliefs that impact their judgment. Sometimes, we need advocates because our own family members may have goals and wishes that differ from ours.

Communication is also an issue. Because of our diminished ability to hear and see, coupled with medical jargon and limited face-to-face time with healthcare providers, we may find it difficult to understand diagnoses and treatment plans. Communication difficulties are further complicated by the disjointed care that happens when multiple specialists are managing chronic conditions. What's more, some treatment options for old people are not covered by insurance, which limit our choices and/or makes treatment unaffordable, a circumstance that an advocate can help us to navigate.

Advocacy is a key factor in ensuring that we get the care we need. Advocates are most often family members such as a spouse, adult children, a sibling or a trusted friend. Your advocate must be willing to put some effort into preparing for the "healthcare interface." He or she must not only understand your goals and needs but must also be the sort who is not intimidated by the doctor's big presence and jargon. Regardless of your choice of advocate, don't assume he or she understands everything about you. This is the time for a serious conversation about what you want and don't want.

Burgess recommends that you and your advocate prepare a written list to help both of you be clear about your concerns and to stay focused. Here are her examples:

- How long will the surgery last?

- Will I be able to see clearly right after the procedure?

- What are the alternatives to this plan?

- Who will be doing the procedure?

- We were planning to go on a short trip next week, should we postpone?

- How long will I need therapy?

- Is this treatment covered by insurance?

- When can I drive?

Also, because it's likely you'll be asked, it's helpful to have with you a list of medications and previous surgeries and diagnoses, especially if the provider is new. These prepared lists save time, do not rely on dimming memory, and help the healthcare team stay focused on the reason for the visit.

Burgess says that "advocacy is taking a leading role in healthcare today," and that its positive impact on healthcare will only grow. Today, she says, it's common to see doctors and nurses using an advocate as a second set of ears as well as for clarification of the care plan. Or the advocate may be included just for providing the patient with the comfort of not being alone. The advocate can even be a professional case manager provided by the healthcare system, or one who is hired by the family or friends.

You'd be extraordinarily lucky to have Bob, a college classmate of mine, as your advocate. He's an MD and keeps up with medicine through journals and updated reference books. If you're a friend in need, his advocacy can go to extreme lengths. Example: His best friend, "Jim," who'd sustained third-degree burns over 30 percent of his body, was hospitalized at a burn unit that was a long drive from Bob's home. Jim not only had burns, but his lungs and kidneys were damaged. To advocate for Jim, Bob drove his RV to a site near the hospital and lived there for three months, spending full days at the hospital. ("It helped," Bob says, "that they recognized my expertise in kidney disease.") Meanwhile, back at home, Bob's wife, Marie, took care of Jim's house and pets. (Marie, who has an impressive background and credentials in nursing, often joins Bob in his advocacy roles.)

With his long view of medicine and the way it's changed over the years, Bob stresses that advocacy has become especially important in light of today's medical environment, in which physicians typically spend fifteen minutes per consultation, or, more likely, the patient will not see the physician at all, but rather the physician's assistant or nurse practitioner. The latter, Bob says, handles 75 percent of the patient load. In addition, physicians are bogged down with "paperwork": computer forms to fill out.

A hospital setting is particularly challenging for both the patient and the advocate. In many hospitals, the patient's GP is not allowed to see his or her patient. Rather, a *hospitalist* becomes the patient's temporary physician. Hospitalists specialize in caring for patients exclusively within a hospital setting, from admission to discharge. They manage a patient's care, coordinating with nurses, specialists, and other healthcare professionals to ensure comprehensive care and earlier detection of problems.

Hospitalists work in shifts. A typical hospitalist schedule is often a seven-on, seven-off schedule. That is, they work seven consecutive 12-hour shifts before having seven days off. In this arrangement, patients may see different doctors, and the doctors have less opportunity to be familiar with their patients. The lack of continuity makes for potential gaps in knowledge about a patient's comprehensive medical history. Not only does this arrangement make for discontinuity of care, but patients feel disconnected from their regular GPs. At the same time, the GPs find their roles diminished, leading to a loss of their acute care skills. For the hospitalist, the high workload can cause stress and burnout.

For Bob to be an advocate at a patient's bedside, he must find out what time the hospitalist is expected to arrive. In preparation for the bedside consultation, he gleans as much information as he can from the charge nurse.

When it's time for the patient to be discharged from the hospital, Bob meets with the discharge personnel to ensure that everyone is clear about follow-up care. This might include a discussion of the patient's home environment, plans for rehabilitation, and the need for caretakers or specialists, such as physical therapists.

Bob even checks on drugs and their dosages, especially after one friend, "Tom," was seriously harmed by an overdose of Gentamicin, an antibiotic that had been given to treat an infection following Tom's hip replacement surgery. Gentamicin, Bob says, "if not properly dosed causes loss of hearing, loss of balance and kidney failure"—all of which happened to Tom. In that case, Bob went beyond advocacy: he was instrumental in getting the surgeon's license revoked for "gross malpractice." As it turned out, several malpractice cases against that surgeon had been previously registered.

In cases where his friends have dementia, in addition to being designated as the advocate, Bob often has durable power of attorney. In these situations, he is present during the initial exam, tests, and treatments. During consultations, he asks questions pertinent to the friend's condition, and makes sure the physician uses simple terms. He also makes suggestions for tests, and at times asks for the rationale for the treatment. He takes notes and makes recordings of every consultation.

In his advocacy work, Bob says he doesn't "directly interfere with the doctor-patient relationship." But he does make it clear that his role is to help both the patient and the physician by presenting a "a clear and unemotional picture of the patient's disease and problems."

Even though you might not have a medical degree, you can do that too—for others as well as for yourself. You can prepare questions ahead of time; take notes and make recordings; and ask the doctor to slow down, repeat unclear statements, and clarify technical terms. As my friend Kristi says, "Advocate, advocate, advocate for yourself, and be demanding on your own behalf."

Part Four: End-of-Life Decisions

Chapter Thirteen

End-of-life care

Hospitals are the default destination for end-of-life care—care that hospitals are typically ill-equipped to handle. The problem is that hospitals are set up to deal with the acutely ill, and the near-death patient is treated the same as a healthier young person. For example, for both the frail old man and the young man with abnormal heart rhythm, the cardiologist suggests an implantable heart device. If no one speaks up, the elderly patient goes to the operating room to receive his device, an option that may be of little value.

Dr. Lydia Dugdale, author of *The Lost Art of Dying*, tells us that the most compelling reason to avoid dying in the hospital is doctors' rescue fantasy. "Doctors are hardwired to free patients from the grip of death, and patients are hardwired to seek safety." The problem is that doctors' rescue efforts can lead to one procedure after another, a situation that may provoke more suffering. In addition, prolonged hospitalization leads to decreased strength for patients as well as to exposure to hospital-acquired infections.

In his book *Being Mortal*, Dr. Gawande says, "As people's capacity wanes, whether through age or ill health, making their lives better often requires curbing our purely medical imperatives—resisting the urge to fiddle and fix and control. But it poses a difficult question: when should we try to fix and when should we not?" That's a tough one. The wise decision is frequently unclear. From my vantage point at this time in my life, I would opt for not fixing (says me with all my surgeries).

Dying in the hospital is extraordinarily expensive: one night in intensive care can easily exceed $10,000. In the United States, 25 percent of all Medicare spending is for the 5 percent of patients who are in their final year of life. Most of that money is used for the patients' last couple of months of life and is of little apparent benefit. Dr. Ashish K. Jha, Professor of Global Health and Health Policy at the Harvard T.H. Chan School of Public Health says, "One way to potentially save money is to reliably predict who will die and therefore would not benefit from receiving intensive care. But this turns out to be extremely hard to do."

Researchers have tried using a sophisticated AI prediction program to identify patients who are most likely to die. They discovered that there is no group of people for whom death is easily predictable. If you can't reliably predict when sick people are going to die, then reducing end-of-life spending becomes extremely difficult. When it's hard to know what will happen, it is hard to know what to do.

Sometimes doctors use frailty assessments to help determine who will benefit from a particular surgery, drug therapy, or hospitalization. Some people are so frail that no good can come of hospitalization. But what about the patients' wishes? I think the patient should be calling the shots—at least that's what I would want to do. But of course, you'd have to be alert enough to make such decisions,

According to the CDC, heart disease is the nation's leading cause of death and disability. It's been diagnosed in more than 18 percent of those over 65. In recent years, dramatic improvements in treatments have helped reduce both heart attacks and cardiac deaths. But because the treatments may not markedly extend the lives of old patients or improve the quality of their remaining years, those treatments are not always the best choice. For example, there's an implantable cardioverter defibrillator (I.C.D.) that delivers a shock in the case of sudden cardiac arrest. Dr. Daniel Matlock, a geriatrician and researcher at the University of Colorado, tells us, "It's easy to sell these things to patients because you say, 'this can prevent sudden cardiac death.' The patient says, 'that sounds great.'" But the intensity of I.C.D. shocks can be severe and can cause anxiety, panic, stress, depression, and even PTSD.

From 2015 through September 2024, surgeons implanted at least 585,000 such devices in patients' chests. But a study of patients whose hearts weren't pumping effectively (but no arteries were blocked), showed that I.C.D.s did not reduce mortality for patients over 70. The devices only prevented sudden cardiac deaths—and those occur more frequently in younger patients. As Dr. Matlock notes, "at 85 or 90, sudden death is not necessarily the worst thing that can happen." Agreed.

Deciding whether someone stands to benefit from dying in the hospital requires facing reality and frank conversations with medical professionals, such as palliative care specialists. Most importantly, it requires the wisdom to discern when enough is enough—when it's time to shift attention from cure to care. Palliative care specialists can help by assessing patients' readiness for tough conversations and then motivating them to prepare for end of life by identifying what they can and cannot control and by prioritizing what matters most.

I have no experience working with such a specialist, but my sister sat through a 30-minute conversation between a dying friend and a palliative care provider who asked questions about pain and daily life. "She was a lovely professional," my sister says, one who provided advice, notes to put on the fridge for 911 responders, and a phone number where she could be reached. "There was no sober, grief stuff."

Sometimes it makes sense to die in the hospital, as in cases when family dynamics prohibit dying well at home, or there's no one to provide sufficient around-the-clock care. Figuring out how to die at home requires planning—not just about acquiring equipment such as a hospital bed, but also organizing family and friends to work shifts.

One in three deaths occurs at home, often with the help of hospice. According to information on a hospice website, the service focuses on the "care, comfort, and quality of life of a person with a serious illness who is approaching the end of life and for whom further treatment is unlikely to be effective." Ideally, hospice programs can provide equipment and medications related to terminal illness as well as a team that may include nurses, doctors, social workers, and home health aides. Hospice also offers emotional and spiritual support, bereavement counseling, and assistance with daily living tasks.

Medicare covers hospice care. Their website says you qualify if you have Medicare Part A (hospital insurance) and meet all of these conditions:

- Your hospice doctor and your regular doctor (if you have one) certify that you're terminally ill (with a life expectancy of 6 months or less).

- You accept comfort care (palliative care) instead of care to cure your illness.

- You sign a statement choosing hospice care instead of other Medicare-covered treatments for your terminal illness and related conditions.

The quality of hospice care varies. As noted by the *Journal of Palliative Medicine*, factors that may contribute to low quality care include "lack of a functioning interdisciplinary team (IDT), minimal physician involvement in direct patient care and clinical IDT meetings, and inadequate responses to symptom emergencies in patients' homes."

According to Dr. Aronson's observations, "the care a patient received increasingly seemed to depend on luck: which nurse was assigned, how busy the hospice was, who was on call during a crisis."

When cardiologist Sandeep Jauhar's father was at the end of his life, Jauhar and his siblings turned to hospice care. They soon discovered, Jauhar writes, a "harsh reality." What they learned, through experience, was that the hospice system "...requires family involvement in the dying process to a degree that even we, as a family of doctors, weren't comfortable with." The family had to handle nearly every aspect of his care. "A nurse was scheduled to come to the house only for about an hour twice a week. Getting an aide to help with basic activities of daily living was nearly impossible." The main problem, Jauhar says, is funding:

> In 2024, the average per-patient Medicare payment to hospice agencies was about $200 a day, with an annual cap of $33,500. That outlay would barely pay for a part-time aide, yet it is also needed to cover medications, medical equipment and nurse visits. So hospice agencies are forced to shift the bulk of responsibilities to families as the dying process unfolds over weeks or months.

By providing so little funding, Dr. Jauhar adds, "...Medicare too often makes hospice care an unviable option." At the same time, hospice has become a multi-billion-dollar, burgeoning industry. Three quarters of hospice agencies are now for-profit, a situation that threatens to put profit maximization over patient well-being. As reported in the *Journal of the American Medical Association*, "Just as private equity acquisition throughout medical specialties has surged in recent years, the hospice industry has been found to be fertile ground for private equity firms. ...Private equity firms see huge profits in buying hospice programs that are providing care for the most vulnerable persons and their families at a sentinel, often tragic time."

Companies maximize profits by decreasing visits by professional staff, using less-skilled people for visits, shifting the cost of expensive medications to Medicare Part D, and enrolling people who are anticipated to have a longer length of stay and less need of intensive hospice services.

The National Hospice and Palliative Care Organization offers resources to help you choose a hospice program. They recommend looking for one that has a not-for-profit status, certification by Medicare, and a long service record. You can compare options by visiting the Medicare Hospice Compare website.

You can also get assistance in end-of-life care by hiring a *death doula*, someone who assists a dying person and their loved ones before, during, and after death. As the Cleveland Clinic website says, "... a death doula provides emotional and physical support, education about the dying process, preparation for what's to come and guidance while you're grieving." Death doulas can provide a variety of services, depending on your needs. For example, they can help oversee end-of-life care, provide guidance in such matters as do-not-resuscitate orders and powers of attorney, assist with obituaries and planning funeral services, provide grief counseling and companionship after someone has died, and find creative ways to honor the person after they've died.

Death doulas are similar to hospice caregivers in that they both offer counseling, spiritual support and other nonmedical services to help a dying person and their loved ones during their final days. But, unlike hospice professionals, death doulas are not licensed to provide hands-on medical assistance. However, they are increasingly becoming an integrated part of hospice care teams. While they are not licensed, death doulas are typically trained and certified. Although there are not yet universally recognized requirements for becoming a death doula, organizations such as the International End-of-Life Doula Association (INELDA) offer training and certification. You can find a death doula at the INELDA website.

Connie Burgess, RN, gave me an excellent end-of-life booklet. It's a fourteen-page guide in large print with clear descriptions about what to expect. It's called "Gone From My Sight: The Dying Experience," by Barbara Karnes, RN. For example, the booklet lists the mental and physical changes you can expect, including those that occur in the days and hours before death. Karnes has dedicated the last 42 years of her life to the education, care, and support of dying people and their loved ones. Her booklets include a five-booklet "end of life guidelines" series. You can find them on the Barbara Karnes website. I was impressed.

As I contemplate various scenarios for the end of my own life, I find I wouldn't choose either dying in a hospital or at home in a drawn-out hospice arrangement with family gathered around. My first choice would be to die from a sudden heart attack as happened with both of my parents. My second choice would be to die by suicide if the quality of my health and life reaches a point that becomes intolerable to me.

Chapter Fourteen

The suicide option

Felicia is the only person I've known who chose to end her own life. Her husband had died of pancreatic cancer, and she had been having TIAs—transient ischemic attacks, in which blood flow to the brain is temporarily disrupted. TIAs are "mini strokes" that usually resolve within minutes or hours. While TIAs are not actual strokes, they are warning signs of a potential future stroke. (There are two kinds of strokes. The most common are ischemic strokes, which are caused by blockages—such as a clot—of an artery. The second are hemorrhagic strokes, which are caused by bleeding, usually as a result of high blood pressure or an aneurysm.)

Felicia decided to end her life rather than risk a stroke. The people who helped her die spoke at her funeral in what I remember was a rather cheerful, upbeat tone. Felicia had joined the Hemlock Society, a right-to-die and assisted suicide advocacy organization. (The organization has since morphed into an organization called Compassion and Choices.) Her death was both peaceful and self-administered—a method referred to as "suicidal asphyxiation by intoxication and plastic bag suffocation." That is, a plastic bag was placed over her head, and helium, from a tank, was used to displace the oxygen in the bag. From what I can gather, such an option is no longer available in the U.S., and such organizations no longer exist.

When I Googled assisted suicide organizations, the first entry that popped up were these words: "You're not alone. Help is available. If you are experiencing difficult thoughts call 988. Emergency number 911." Moving on, I did find "right to die" advocacy groups. These organizations, including Compassion and Choices, promote medical aid in dying laws (the term "physician-assisted suicide" is no longer used). The common acronym for medical aid in dying, which I'm seeing more often, is MAID. At the time of this writing, eleven states plus the District of Columbia have enacted such laws. The practice has also been legalized in nine countries on three continents.

To qualify for MAID in the U.S., you must be at least 18 years old; have a terminal disease with less than six months to live; have the mental capacity to request aid in dying; be a resident of a state where such a law is in effect; and be capable of making and communicating your own healthcare decisions. You must also be able to be able to talk well enough to be understood, swallow what the doctor prescribes without assistance, hold a glass, and mix the drink on your own. Depending on where you live, you may be able to choose between administering the drug yourself or having a healthcare provider inject a drug that stops your heart. In some states, you must also be able to get yourself into a pharmacy to purchase the lethal prescription. All states, except Oregon and Vermont, require that you reside in the state where MAID is offered. Because Felicia didn't have a terminal illness, she wouldn't have qualified for MAID.

Amy Bloom, author of *In Love: A Memoir of Love and Loss*, writes of her experience in helping her husband, Brian Ameche, end his life. At the age of 67, he had been diagnosed with Alzheimer's disease and had decided that the "long goodbye," as that disease is commonly characterized, was not for him. Like Felicia, Brian wouldn't qualify for physician-assisted suicide. As Bloom writes, "Right to die in America is about as meaningful as the right to eat or the right to decent housing; you've got the right, but it doesn't mean you're going to get the goods."

Brian left it to Amy to choose the best method for ending his life. Because she did the research and has enumerated the results in her book, I have used it as my primary resource for this chapter. Before listing the suicide options researched by Bloom, I'll tell you that, ultimately, she chose an organization in Switzerland called Dignitas, which she describes as "the only place in the world for painless, peaceful, and legal suicide." More on that later.

Her investigation led to consideration of the following methods:

Drowning: When Amy suggests it, Brian responds, "Are you kidding me? It's cold. No."

Voluntary suspension of eating and drinking (VSED): Recommended by some groups as the only effective, legal, and certain end to life. But it can take weeks. A doctor Amy interviews tells her it's not easy, and then asks, "How big's your husband?" (Note: Samuel Harrington, MD, author of *At Peace: Choosing a Good Death After a Long Life*, writes, "the refusal of fluid and food is an effective and ethical option...," noting also that death is by dehydration, not starvation, and that most patients will die in six to ten days, and 85 percent will have passed away quietly within two weeks. He also writes that people experience "a sense of euphoria that rapidly displaces most sensations of hunger.")

Phenobarbital: For a large-enough dose, you can possibly get it from "not-too-fussy" veterinarians in Mexico; otherwise, a large-enough dose is difficult to get in the U.S., unless you can "find a vet who will believe you have a horse you wish to put down."

Sodium pentobarbital: A sedative that will kill you painlessly in less than a minute. But it takes a lethal dose, of course. It's what's used in lethal injections for executions. The pills come in fifty- or one-hundred-milligram tablets, but Bloom needs five hundred (20 grams). She manages to convince a doctor that she needs it for her intractable insomnia. But all the pharmacies she contacts let her know that they'd never be able to get it for her.

Carbon monoxide poisoning: In which you sit in your car with the engine running and a hose connecting the tailpipe to the inside of the car. Apparently, this has been made difficult because catalytic converters reduce CO emissions from cars. Also, this method requires a garage, which Amy doesn't have. A friend offers her garage.

She also considers street drugs but worries about their dependability.

Bloom was warned not to search for suicide methods on the internet, in case Brian's death looks suspicious. In the same vein, she notes that, if she were to assist in his suicide, she'd have to wear gloves so her fingerprints cannot be found on, say, a blender in which she has made a phenobarbital-laced smoothie.

Bloom finally settles on Dignitas, a Swiss nonprofit organization, which, for 20 years, has been offering "accompanied suicide." (Switzerland legalized assisted suicide in 1942.) Before Dignitas agrees to assist Brian, there is much to be done, including a multitude of forms to submit. Bloom must prove that she would not gain any financial benefit from Brian's death. Brian must write a biography and essay about why he wants an accompanied suicide. Other required documents include birth certificate, divorce papers, marriage certificate, and even dental records so that the Swiss police can identify his body. Two physicians must provide documents showing that Brian is mentally competent with sound judgment, with no hint that he's suffering from depression. The cost is $10,000.

After arriving in Switzerland, a doctor from Dignitas conducts two interviews to assess Brian's discernment and determination. At this point, Brian is considered to be on his way to the "provisional green light." (It turns out that 70 percent of the people who get the provisional green light never contact Dignitas again; they just want reassurance that the option is open.) After getting the green light, a Swiss doctor writes the prescription for the sodium pentobarbital that Brian drinks at the final appointment, which happens at an apartment in Zurich.

Daniel Kahneman, Nobel laureate and author of the international best seller, *Thinking, Fast and Slow*, also chose to end his life using Dignitas services. He was 90 and in reasonably good health. Explaining his decision to podcasters Katarzyna de Lazari-Radek and Peter Singer, he wrote, "I have believed since I was a teenager that the miseries and indignities of the last years of life are superfluous, and I am acting on that belief. I am still active, enjoying many things in life (except the daily news) and will die a happy man. But my kidneys are on their last legs, the frequency of mental lapses is increasing, and I am 90 years old. It is time to go." He believed that if he did not end his life when he was clearly mentally competent, he could lose control over the remainder of it and live and die with "needless miseries and indignities."

In Oregon, the first state to legalize medical aid in dying for the terminally ill, people report that they have chosen that option for the following reasons: Losing autonomy (89 percent); being less able to engage in activities that make life enjoyable (88 percent); loss of dignity (64 percent); feeling like a burden (42 percent).

Britain recently approved plans to legalize assisted suicide. As of July 2025, it had not yet become law, but, if passed, it will join more than a dozen jurisdictions that permit medically assisted aid in dying. In 2002, the Netherlands became the first country to add MAID to their universal health system offerings. In 2024, nearly 10,000 people in that country (5 percent of deaths) chose that option.

When Canada introduced its Medical Assistance in Dying program in 2016, it was available only to adults suffering from an incurable and intolerable disease and whose death was "reasonably foreseeable." In 2021, the reasonably foreseeable requirement was removed, thus legalizing MAID for people suffering from such conditions as chronic pain and certain neurological disorders. Since 2021, the young, the poor, and the desperate are choosing state-facilitated death. Canada has become the world's fastest-growing euthanasia regime, with MAID now accounting for about one in 20 deaths—63,000 as of 2023. The central principle of Canada's stance on euthanasia is autonomy—honoring a patient's wishes to be in control.

In Colombia, Spain, Ecuador and the Canadian province of Quebec, people who have been diagnosed with Alzheimer's disease or other kinds of dementia can apply for an advance request for assisted death while they are still able to consent for themselves. That leaves someone else in the position of making the decision to end that person's life. Who should that person be?

In an op-ed article for *The New York Times*, Journalist Louise Perry, a native of Britain, notes that "every one of these jurisdictions [countries that have legalized MAID] has a total fertility rate below the replacement threshold. I do not think this is a coincidence. The state, with its almighty power, is tasked with both paying for the support of the old and disabled and regulating their dying." Encouraging citizens to accept MAID, Perry suggests, looks like a cost-saving measure at a time when the financial burden of caring for old people has never been greater. "The moral peril is greatest in countries like mine," Perry says, "in which a socialized health care and pension system has a strong incentive to winnow out its most expensive users." From a financial perspective in Britain, the only problem with MAID programs is that they seem "too popular among the young and insufficiently popular among the old."

But they can save the state a good deal of money: research has predicted that MAID could save Canada $34.7 to $138.8 million in annual health care spending. The British government forecasts that the government could save tens of millions of pounds per year, once the program is adopted.

Perry doesn't believe that assisted suicide should be legalized. But if it is, she thinks the state shouldn't be party to it. At the same time, countries, such as the U.K., that have government-funded health care, must figure out how to pay medical expenses for old people from their ever-dwindling coffers.

Perry fears that allowing governments to be party to assisted suicide would lead them to be "inexorably tugged toward what looks to a mindless bureaucracy like a 'solution'"—a reference to the Holocaust. To keep the government out of it, Perry thinks that "the best system to emulate is the one adopted by Switzerland, in which patients are legally helped to die through nonprofit organizations independent of the state." That, of course, is Dignitas.

According to Perry, the largely privatized American healthcare system, for all its problems, is less motivated to winnow down its most expensive users than countries with socialized medicine. Those costly users, of course, are us old people. That is, we're not being persuaded by our healthcare providers to save taxpayer money by forgoing possible life-saving expensive treatments. Instead, the more treatments we get, the more money is made by our profit-driven corporate healthcare enterprises. (During the Covid epidemic, when elective surgeries plummeted, hospitals needed massive infusions of government funding to survive.)

This is something I'd never thought about: suicide as a money-saver. Savings aside, I think medically-assisted suicide is a reasonable end-of-life option—even for those whose deaths from disease are not imminent. But how do you regulate it?

Chapter Fifteen

Disposing of your dead body

Since you're not going to live forever, you might as well make a plan for disposing of your dead body. I'm a fan of Caitlin Doughty. She's a mortician based in L.A. and author of *Smoke Gets in Your Eyes*, about working in a crematorium, and *From Here to Eternity*, about how other nations and cultures deal with death. She's a funny lady, a good writer, and an advocate for funeral industry reform. Much of the information in this chapter comes from her books.

In America, death has been a big business since the turn of the twentieth century. America's funeral industry has become more expensive, more corporate, and more bureaucratic than any other funeral industry on earth. (American funerals cost $8,000 to $10,000, not including the burial plot and cemetery costs.) What's more, our funeral system is notorious for passing laws and regulations to interfere with diverse death practices and for enforcing conformity to Americanized norms. After Hurricane Katrina, a group of Benedictine monks in southern Louisiana began selling low-cost, handmade cypress caskets. The state's Board of Embalmers and Funeral Directors drummed up a cease-and-desist order, claiming that only funeral homes licensed by their board could sell "funeral merchandise." (Eventually, a federal judge sided with the monks.)

An executive of Service Corporation International, the country's largest funeral and cemetery company, admitted that "the industry was really built around selling a casket." As more of us are choosing cremations, the funeral industry must find new ways to survive financially.

Many Muslims would like to be able to open funeral homes in the United States. Muslims reject embalming and recoil at the idea of cutting into the body and injecting it with chemicals and preservatives. The Islamic custom is to wash and purify the body immediately after death, then bury it as quickly as possible, ideally before nightfall. Yet many states have heavy-handed regulations that require funeral homes to *offer* embalming and for all funeral directors to be trained as embalmers, even though the embalming process itself is never required. Obviously, in states with such regulations, Muslims would be prohibited from opening funeral homes.

Most people choose either traditional burials or cremation. But neither one of these choices is earth friendly. The problem with traditional burials—that is, an embalmed body placed in a casket—are the heaps of toxic materials that go into the ground: 4.3 million gallons of embalming fluids; 1.6 million tons of reinforced concrete; 17,000 tons of copper and bronze; 64,000 tons of steel. Traditional burials are also the most expensive: the median price of a funeral with burial in 2023 was about $10,000, *not including* the cemetery plot or a monument.

Cremations now account for nearly two-thirds of body disposals in the U.S. But cremations are also ecologically problematic: The cremation process uses the same amount of energy required for a 500-mile car trip—roughly the same amount of energy as a single person uses in an entire month. Also, cremation releases 400 Kgs of carbon dioxide into the atmosphere plus a host of other pollutants and carcinogens, the worst of which is mercury from dental fillings.

If you want to avoid both traditional burial and cremation, you might be able to arrange a green burial. A green burial is one in which they wrap your body in a cloth or put it in a biodegradable container and bury you in the ground. (You can also choose a coffin made of mushroom mycelium, which decomposes within 30 to 45 days. Similarly, your body can be put in a mushroom burial suit, in which mushroom spores are sewn into the fabric. The spores help decompose your body.)

The trick to arranging a green burial is finding a cemetery that allows this. Paula Span, writing in *The New York Times*, has purchased a cemetery plot in Wellfleet, Massachusetts, that allows green burials. Perhaps such burials are becoming more popular. When she asked the town cemetery commissioner, "Do you see a lot of interest in green burials?" the commissioner replied, "I don't think we've had a traditional burial in two years. It's all green." A small industry has evolved to produce artisanal woven caskets, linen shrouds, and other eco-friendly funerary items.

The first cemetery that allowed green burials was Ramsey Creek Preserve in Westminster, South Carolina, in 1998. By 2016, the number of green burial cemeteries had increased to 150. In 2025, 497 cemeteries were offering green burials. By the time you read this, the numbers will surely have increased. Most cemeteries that allow green burials are hybrids. That is, they accommodate both conventional and green burials. Some cemeteries are dedicated exclusively to green burials, and some operate in partnership with land trusts, such as the Nature Conservancy.

Using Google, I found nine green burial cemeteries in California, my home state. One of these is in Joshua Tree National Park. Its website describes their process, one that I found interesting enough to include here:

Joshua Tree Memorial Park's Natural Burial sections are located in an "open desert" area on the property adjacent to our traditional burial garden sites. Graves are hand dug using shovels, pick axes, and pry bars by 2 or 3 grounds crew members.

The digging can take anywhere from 7-10 hours depending on the hardness of the ground. The grave is dug to a 5-foot depth on average. The Green Burial Council's recommended depth is 3.5 feet. A minimum distance of 18 inches is needed to keep the body out of the "smell zone"—the distance between the deceased and the surface that makes the odor noticeable to humans or other animal species.

Grave spots measure 10' long and 5' wide, on average. The inner box of the grave space measures 8' long and 3' wide. Before the digging is started, native plants are temporarily removed from the area.

The deceased is transported to the site either in its organic casket or other container or, when the body is shrouded, on a wood carrying board. The body (along with any bio-degradable receptacle) is placed on a standard lowering device.

Once in the ground, the body is covered with a two-foot layer of dirt. Medium to large rocks are collected from the surrounding desert and a layer of these stones are added into the burial site. This is done for a variety of reasons. Firstly, to create a deterrent barrier against any local wildlife that may attempt to dig into the grave. Secondly, to create a reference point for the depth of the grave if it is ever probed to determine location. Thirdly, to add stability to the grave site. After the rock layer is added, the hole's remaining open space is filled in with dirt. Any plants removed from the site are added back to location.

Traditional memorialization, such as granite or bronze grave markers and headstones, are not allowed in the natural burial sections. To mark the site, families may use a large rock—with minimal decoration—or plant a naturally occurring plant (native to the Joshua Tree area).

Unfortunately, burial in your back yard isn't usually allowed, although in rare cases—through a process involving numerous permits—it might be possible.

Composting is becoming an increasingly popular body disposal option. In this process, your body is put into a steel cylinder (compost bin!) along with soil, wood chips, alfalfa, and straw. After several weeks, it turns into about 300 pounds of soil that family members can use for planting or donate to a local land conservancy. As of this writing, twelve states have passed laws to allow human composting: Washington (the first to legalize), Colorado, Maine, Oregon, California, Minnesota, Delaware, Maryland, Arizona, Nevada, New York, and Vermont.

As with composting, a process called *alkaline hydrolysis—or aquamation*—uses a large container to break your body down into its chemical components. The container is a sort of pressure cooker that's filled with water and potassium hydroxide and heated to 320 degrees. In about four to six hours, your body is reduced to bone and liquid. Bone fragments are rinsed and pulverized to dust ("ash") and placed in an urn. (Wikipedia tells me that Benjamin Tutu was "aquamated" per his wish in South Africa.) At this writing, 29 states allow alkaline hydrolysis.

If you live near the ocean, you can have your body dumped there. Here's an example of full-body sea burial offered by a service near my home. The price starts at $4,800. The boat can take up to 35 passengers. Because the ocean is, as they say, "a very fragile ecosystem," bodies are either shrouded in cotton or placed in an "eco-friendly wicker or natural fiber casket," and natural rock or sand is used to weight the body. They won't take embalmed bodies or bodies that are "actively participating in or recently took part in chemotherapy." The burial takes four hours. Of course, you can also scatter ashes at sea. The starting price for that is $375.

If you live in Saguache County, Colorado, you can be cremated in a fire through the services of the Crestone End of Life Project. The process involves a pyre, a half-cord of wood, a wooden stretcher and a shroud. As far as I know, this is the only place in the U.S. that allows cremation in an outdoor pyre. You must be a resident of the county to use its services. In the "testimonials" section of their website, I read the following: "What a beautiful way to go, on an altar, in the open air, on the side of a mountain..." and, "That was the most amazing, loving and spiritual gathering/ceremony/send-off for John, a wonderful person honored by wonderful people in a wonderful, heart-centered ceremony in an awesome space!"

Because we have learned of the environmental consequences of cremation, my husband and I have opted to have our bodies composted. That option—called "natural organic reduction"—was recently legalized in California. The law does not go into effect until 2027, allowing for regulations to be hammered out. Nevertheless, at this writing, in 2026, it appears that at least one company is ready to sign people up: A friend of mine recently received a brochure advertising its "pre-planning" services for an "eco-friendly alternative to cremation." The title of the brochure is "Understanding Soil Transformation."

I think my husband and I can probably hang on a couple of more years until California's natural organic reduction law goes into effect.

Final Word: Older and wiser?

I've been wracking my brain trying to think of something wise to say. The common expression, "older and wiser," implies that we old people automatically become wise because of the experiences and knowledge we've acquired over the course of our long lives. It's true that we have had more time to accumulate experiences, although I'm not sure that makes us wise. We do have the long view, but does that make us wiser than younger people?

I was born during Franklin Delano Roosevelt's first term. I can remember the Second World War, but not the horrors of it. What I remember is a child's eye view, such as going around the neighborhood collecting grease for the war effort. Grease, such as bacon fat, was turned into glycerin which was turned into explosives. We also collected tinfoil, painstakingly separating the foil from the paper backing of gum wrappers we might find in a gutter. We'd roll the foil into balls which were then shredded into flakes and dropped from aircraft into enemy airspace, causing radar-controlled weapons to miss their targets. As a child, I had no idea what these materials were used for, just that they were for "the war effort."

Some things were better in the "old days." I'm glad I was raised before the advent of digital devices, or even of television (my family bought one when

I was 16). I'm glad to have been a "free range" kid, living the unsupervised life, riding my bike to school, playing outside with neighbor kids all day. I'm glad that, if I were sick, the doctor would come to my house.

My dad, whose formal education ended in the tenth grade, was born in Russia and emigrated to the United States when he was five. He worked at Sears for 18 years, then took advantage of their profit-sharing plan to open a clothing store for boys. (Sears, one of the largest retailers in the country, filed for bankruptcy in 2018. Old people will remember their mail-order catalogue—the "wish book" of its day.)

My mother, whose formal education ended in the seventh grade, was born in Austria and emigrated to the United States at age four. She went to secretarial school in Los Angeles and got a job with a title company, which she enjoyed. After marriage and children, she became a homemaker, as was expected in those days (also expected when I married in the late 1950s). She did a good job at housekeeping but also needed to channel her talents and skills by attaining leadership positions in civic organizations, including PTA (president), Girl Scouts (commissioner), and La Casa (I forget her role), a community center in our town that provided educational and social services. (The organization was founded in 1946 and is still operating.)

Our home in the Los Angeles suburbs had two bedrooms and one bath. We had two cars. My sister and I both attended a private college, which cost $750 a semester, for tuition, board and room. I'm only mentioning these niceties because the middle-class opportunities we enjoyed are no longer possible for a family whose breadwinner's education ends in tenth grade and who works as a department store salesperson—or even manager. According to experts, income inequality has been rising steadily for 50 years and keeps getting worse. The highest-earning 20 percent of Americans continue to capture a disproportionate share of total income compared to middle- and lower-income families.

But some things are better now, especially some aspects of individual freedom. In our part of the world, gay people can be themselves, women can achieve as much or more than men, Black people have moved to the forefront of culture, civic life, and leadership. Since 1936, the year I was born, life expectancy has increased from about 60 to nearly 80 years.

As I look back over my long life, I find that I still can't offer any words of wisdom. Maybe some old people can. I wondered if there is any truth to the "older and wiser" notion, so I did a Google search and found that academics have made a study of wisdom. Their definitions of wisdom are all over the place.

One says wisdom is maintaining a sense of positive well-being and kindness in the face of challenges. Another tells us that "Wise people are able to accept reality as it is, with equanimity," and that old people who tested high on the wisdom measurement scale were more likely to have better coping skills. For example, they'd be more active than passive about dealing with hardship.

Other academics tell us that wisdom is characterized by a reduction in self-centeredness; that wise people try to understand situations from multiple perspectives, not just their own. As a result, we become tolerant. "You're not only regulating your emotional state, you're also attending to another person's emotional state. You're not focusing so much on what you need and deserve, but on what you can contribute."

An octogenarian psychotherapist says that acceptance of aging is necessary for growth, but "it's not a resigned acceptance; it's an embracing acceptance." A tall order, I think.

Erik Erikson (1902-1994), a pioneering psychologist known for his groundbreaking theory of development, defined eight stages of human development, arguing that personality develops throughout our lifespans, with each stage building upon the previous one. (He coined the term "identity crisis.") The eight stages are:

1. Infancy: Trust versus mistrust. Infants develop a sense of trust if their needs are consistently met, leading to a feeling of security. If needs are not met, mistrust and fear may develop.

2. Early childhood: Autonomy versus shame and doubt. Children begin to assert their independence and self-control, either developing a sense of autonomy or feeling ashamed and doubtful of their abilities.

3. Preschool: Initiative versus guilt. Children begin to initiate activities and take the lead, either developing a sense of initiative or feeling guilty about their actions.

4. School age: Industry versus inferiority. Children strive to develop competence in new skills, either developing a sense of industry or feeling inferior compared to peers.

5. Adolescence: Identity versus role confusion. Adolescents explore different roles and identities, either developing a sense of self or experiencing role confusion.

6. Young adulthood: Intimacy versus isolation. Young adults try to form intimate relationships with others, either developing a sense of intimacy or feeling isolated.

7. Middle adulthood: Generativity versus stagnation. Adults are either concerned for and committed to contributing to the next generation and society, or they feel stagnant.

8. Late adulthood: Integrity versus despair. Older adults reflect on
their lives, either developing a sense of "ego integrity," believing
that they've had a fulfilling and meaningful life, or feeling despair
because of regrets about their past.

When he was in his 80s, Erikson found a need to add a ninth stage of
development. Along with his wife, Joan, he re-examined the eight stages
and concluded that we might find that old people have reverted to the less
desirable outcomes of the stages. For example, an old person may become
mistrustful, as described in stage one's trust versus mistrust. The Eriksons
found that we old people are more likely to develop a positive perspective about life if we've come to terms with the changes and adjustments
required of us. At the same time, they believe that when old people lack
challenges, self-absorption and stagnation may take over. The key, they say,
is to set goals that match our current capacities.

Some people suggest that sliding into the "old old" category leads us
into some of the stages of grief proposed by Elizabeth Kubler- Ross. First,
we're in denial, as in refusing to acknowledge our newly acquired deficits.
(That's me.) The bargaining stage might look like the efforts we make, such
as exercise, or dyeing our hair, to maintain some semblance of our younger
selves. (Exercise, yes; dyed hair, no.) For some, Kubler-Ross's "anger" and
"depression" stages come into play. (Not me.) Eventually, we may reach
the acceptance phase, some sooner than others. (I might be getting there.
My sister reports that she seems to waver between acceptance and self-pity,
depending on her health and social opportunities.)

I like Ursula M. Staudinger's definition of wisdom and think it's closest
to what I consider the truth. Staudinger is a "lifespan psychologist" and
professor at Columbia University. She says that personal wisdom involves
five elements: "self-insight; the ability to demonstrate personal growth;

self-awareness in terms of your historical era and your family history; understanding that priorities and values, including your own, are not absolute; and an awareness of life's ambiguities."

True wisdom, Staudinger tells us, involves recognizing the negative both within and outside ourselves and trying to learn from it. She believes that wisdom, as she has defined it, is extremely rare and that, in fact, it declines in our final decades. We're more likely to look back on our lives and say that the events that occurred were for the best. A wise person, she says, would acknowledge mistakes and losses and still try to improve. Trying to be positive about life when we're older is a coping strategy.

In sum: I don't think old people are wiser than anyone else.

As I struggled to come up with words of wisdom, odds and ends of aphorisms popped into my head:

> From a Girl Scouts song: "Make new friends, but keep the old, one is silver and the other is gold." (It can be sung in a round.)

> Or, from the Bible: "Do unto others as you would have them do unto you." (Why do so few people practice this?)

> Finally, from Yogi Berra: "You should always go to other people's funerals, otherwise they won't come to yours."

That's the best I can do.

Acknowledgements

First thanks go to my first reviewers: husband Speed Leas, sister Elaine Jordan, and friend Betsy Wootten. Their suggested additions and changes helped to set me on the right path. Special thanks to Betsy, a skilled proofreader who spared me the embarrassment of typos and grammatical errors. If you find any, they're probably from my later additions.

I'm particularly indebted to Anne Janzer, a nonfiction book coach, who took an interest in my project and helped with innumerable suggestions for improving the book. Lucky for me, she lives in a nearby town. We've become friends.

Special thanks to my daughter, Jocelyn, for creating the book cover artwork.

I'm also grateful for my "village" of contributors whose lived experiences of dealing with old age—both their own and those of people they care for—provide the real world illustrations of our new realities. To begin with, I must thank my (older!) sister Elaine, whose stories and comments are peppered throughout the book.

Here's the rest of the village and the chapters where you'll find them:

Falling: William and Sarah Klair

Exercise: Donna Love, George Killingsworth, Susan Hancey, Michelle Jensen

Living Arrangements: Janet Vandevender, Zeva Lahorgue, Donna Smith, Nick Piediscalzi, Kim Brown, Lanna Giles Tanzi
Caregiving: Cheryl Berry, Mary Leas Stegall, Alice Kelly
Advocacy: Connie Burgess, RN, and Bob Austin, MD

Bibliography

Aronson, Louise. *Elderhood: Redefining Aging, Transforming Medicine, Reimagining Life*. Bloomsbury Adult, 2021.

Attia, Peter, MD, Gifford, Bill. *Outlive: The Science and Art of Longevity*. Harmony, 2023.

Bloom, Amy. *In Love: A Memoir of Love and Loss*. Random House. 2023.

Doughty, Caitlin. *Smoke Gets in Your Eyes: And Other Lessons from the Crematory*. W.W. Norton & Company, 2014.

___*From Here to Eternity: Traveling the World to Find a Good Death*. W.W. Norton & Company, 2017.

___*Will My Cat Eat My Eyeballs: And Other Questions About Dead Bodies*. W.W. Norton & Company, 2020.

Douthat, Ross. *The Deep Places: A memoir of Illness and Discovery*. Convergent Books. 2021.

Dugdale, L.S. *The Lost Art of Dying: Reviving Forgotten Wisdom*. HarperOne, 2021.

Englehart, Katie. *The Inevitable: Dispatches on the Right to Die*. Griffin, 2022.

Gawande, Atul. *Being Mortal: Medicine and What Matters in the End*. New York: Metropolitan Books. Henry Holt and Company, 2014.

Grierson, Bruce. *What Makes Olga Run?: The Mystery of the 90-Something Track Star and What She Can Teach Us About Living Longer, Happier Lives*. St. Martin's Griffin, 2015.

Harrington, Samuel. *At Peace: Choosing a Good Death After a Long Life*. Balance, 2018.

Harris, Ian. *Surgery, The Ultimate Placebo*. Newsouth, 2016.

Kay, Adam. *Undoctored*. Trapeze, 2024.

Locker, George. *Falling Is Not an Option: A Way to Lifelong Balance*. BookBaby, 2020.

Morris, Virginia. *How to Care for Aging Parents: A One-Stop Resource for All Your Medical, Financial, Housing, and Emotional Issues*. Third edition. Workman Publishing Company, 2014.

Offit, Paul. *Overkill: When Modern Medicine Goes Too Far*. Harper Paperbacks, 2022.

Ramakrishnan, Venki. *Why We Die: The New Science of Aging and the Quest for Immortality*. William Morrow, 2025.

Sheehy, Gail. *Passages in Caregiving: Turning Chaos into Confidence*. William Morrow, 2011.

Shepherd, Richard. *The Seven Ages of Death*. Penguin, 2023.

Thomas, Elizabeth Marshall. *Growing Old: Notes on Aging with Something Like Grace*. SanFran, 2021.